SLENDER ME NATURALLY

by
Bernard Jensen, Ph.D.

THE INFORMATION PRESENTED HERE WAS GATHERED DURING OVER 50 YEARS OF SANITARIUM EXPERIENCE, WORKING WITH DIET, EXERCISE AND THE NATURAL HEALING ART TO BRING PATIENTS TO A RIGHT WAY OF LIVING, A RIGHT WEIGHT AND A RIGHT OUTLOOK.

GW00569904

Cover design by Frank Morton, Third Planet Design

PUBLISHED BY: Bernard Jensen, Ph.D.
Route 1, Box 52
Escondido, CA 92025

First Edition

Copyright 1986 Bernard Jensen
ALL RIGHTS RESERVED

BERNARD JENSEN, Publisher
Route 1, Box 52
Escondido, CA 92025

ISBN 0-932615-00-7

Dedication

*To the human body that has the possibility for change
to beauty and good health through discipline and willpower
and TO THE POTENTIAL THAT LIES WITHIN YOU.*

CONTENTS

Foreword

As I see it, overweight equals a state of disharmony, a sign that we haven't come into our real self. In my sanitarium work, I treat obesity as if it were a disease—and, in fact, many times, obesity may either be caused by a disease, or, conversely, may itself result in a disease, contributing to a host of potential problems in the body.

We find that a disease can result in a poor metabolism so that we cannot break down the fat. The liver can be at fault. The pancreas can be underfunctioning, not taking care of the starches and sugars. There is a possibility we are not getting enough oxygen. A underactive thyroid can be responsible in this case. The circulation can be poor.

Possibly it comes back to simple things such as the kitchen table being responsible for an overweight condition. It may be that our environment isn't good. Pollution can cause trouble, especially when fumes, gases, odors and so forth affect the thyroid gland and trigger imbalance in the metabolism, producing a lack of oxygenation. Of course, oxygenation is needed for burning up the fatty tissue in the body. We have to look at the diet, we have to look at the lifestyle, we have to look at the mentality and attitude, we have to look at diseases that may be contributing to obesity or overweight. So we have many things to consider. This is why we have to look at obesity as a disease.

As far as how obesity contributes to the malfunctioning of the human body, the ways are myriad. They include the physiological symptoms such as: high blood pressure, atherosclerosis, arteriosclerosis, diabetes and venous congestion. In addition, however, there are many indirect physical and psychological impacts upon the person carrying too many excess pounds. The obese person is really a well-nourished person—most often it is unchecked preferences for high-calorie, low-nutrition foods or a poorly balanced diet that have contributed to this state. This calorie-stuffed, vitamin-and-mineral deficient individual is rarely a happy person either. Not only does the person's own self esteem suffer from the knowledge that his or her potential is going unattained, but also, there is great external pressure from a society that places increasing emphasis on looking and acting trim, fit and youthful.

I cannot promise eternal youth, of course, but I can offer a new vitality, increased energy and the joy of a better-functioning body at its correct weight to anyone who is willing to read carefully, to take me seriously and to exercise the self control required to break old habits and establish a new healthful lifestyle. Happily, the "willpower" phase is relatively brief—again and again my patients report that as they begin to treat their bodies kindly with proper nutrition and exercise, they no longer crave the foods that formerly were their downfall.

In this book, my goal is to give you some basic concepts of nutrition, exercise and overall good health. Plus the motivation to apply this knowledge at home. According to studies done by various universities, at least 42% of the people in the U.S. qualify as obese (normally defined as being 20% or more over the weight that would be correct for a person's height and frame.) Impersonal statistics aside, the one great need I see is that I must take care of the patient on the other end of the end of the symptoms.

Now, of course, it is sometimes very difficult to teach a person to watch calories carefully and exercise regularly. I would say that 70% of the patients who are overweight need to learn these things. This is where this book is really going to be of value to the average person.

The average person should recognize that we cannot solve the basic problem of overweight with drugs or surgery. There are all kinds of doctoring methods applied today to overcoming obesity. We have people who are taking pills. They want to go the easiest way. One of my patients was a doctor who wanted to reduce weight without changing his habits of living. He weighed something like 250 pounds and he told me, "I'll wait until they make food out of sawdust so I won't gain any weight." Well, he is still waiting. This is pure proscrastination.

Looking at overweight as a chronic disease, a chronic condition, we find it comes on little by little. The overweight condition developed because of transgressing certain natural laws. In this book, we're trying to get you to see these laws from a diet standpoint, even from a psychological standpoint. We find that the psychologist today is doing a lot of good work just by taking care of the mind of a person, and losing weight is both a mental and physical exercise. On the mental side, we have to consider the home environment, the family situation and relationships, the person's attitude. What cultural or other learned food preferences does this person have? How much change is this person willing to make for the sake of becoming slender and energetic?

Because most people gain weight pleasurably at the table, they have not been prodded to seek professional help because of pains, aches or other usual symptoms of dysfunction. The pounds creep on, almost unnoticed, until, one day, you realize there are no notches left to let out your belt, your clothes have all "shrunk" beyond wearability, you're too tired, too short of breath to really enjoy the exercise you know you need, and the road back to slenderness begins to look long indeed.

On the physical side, we have to consider diet, body chemistry, circulation, exercise. Above all, I would say that 70% of the potential for successful weight control depends on the patient's attitude toward this process. It is impossible to give a patient a pill, a "magic bullet" for a fast cure. You worked your way into this trouble, as a rule, and you will have to work your way out of it. As they return to a natural weight, they go through an adjustment period and this is not always pleasant. We have to consider that such an adjustment period may be coming.

But there is hope. As far as testimonials are concerned, I could tell you about Dolly Dimple of circus fame who once weighed 555 pounds. I can show you the pictures of her first as a circus fat lady and they as she looked after going through my reducing diet until she weighed only 118 pounds. I can tell you about our own office employees who took hold of some of these ideas. One of the girls lost 50 pounds and another 20 pounds. I see this sort of thing happening every day. I want to encourage you to follow a good philosophy for handling your life. Without a good philosophy, you cannot be slender. You may find problems in your work. You might find problems in your marriage. You might find your lilfestyle produces stress and strain. These may be contributing to overeating. You need a philosophy that guides you, one that is going to help you with these things.

This book is put together with the idea that the best path for the most people is the middle way. I have tried to show you what to watch out for. I have tried to tell you that successful weight-loss dieting requires patience and persistence. I recommend that you stay on the health side as much as possible.

Now, in my book, I am trying to show you that when you succeed in losing weight with a good reducing diet, then you should follow it up with a healthy way of living *to keep your weight down.* You should know that most reducing diets are not complete. They cannot build a whole body because they are one-sided diets, lacking in nutrients we need. My diet is balanced to meet all nutritional needs while you are losing weight, and I introduce exercise plans and many lifestyle tips to maintain a healthy way of life during and after your weight loss goal is reached.

There are specific people who have to have supervision. It doesn't work for everyone just to go off on their own. Some dieting measures are harmful, and you have to make sure you are not following a dangerous diet. Sometimes to overcome what happens due to extreme diets is a very difficult thing. We know those people who have gotten into anorexia nervosa and bulimia are difficult to handle. It sometimes takes the supervision and experience of a doctor who has handled these kinds of cases. I urge anyone with a health condition to consult a doctor before beginning this or any diet and exercise program. Certain conditions may be aggravated by even a well-balanced nutritional program.

I want to tell you that resolving your weight problem is a way of enlightenment if you follow the path presented in this book. You will feel good, look good and like the way you look and feel, enough to be motivated to stay on the path of harmony, the path of health, the path of right living. You can tell yourself, this is the way to *Slender Me, Naturally!*

Introduction

"A New You"

There are so many books, pills and powders out these days promising quick and easy weight loss that the average person tends to be confused about the right way to lose excess weight. In over 50 years of sanitarium practice, I have helped hundreds of overweight men and women grow slender without drugs or reducing powders, and this was accomplished without actually focusing on weight reduction. How? By introducing them to a more natural way of living.

The key to weight control is not dieting but **lifestyle**. Nutrition, exercise, rest, fresh air, sunshine, recreation, work and relationships all affect our state of well-being, and our body weight molds to those things. When I teach a patient how to change to a healthier, more natural lifestyle, and the patient follows my program faithfully, body weight normalizes. That is, overweight persons tend to lose weight, while underweight persons tend to gain. We find that nature knows best, but sometimes we have to give her a helping hand.

Most people do not realize that a balanced weight control program must be learned, just as we would learn to play the piano. During the first few practice sessions, we can expect to hit a few sour notes. It is normal to make mistakes in learning a new skill, and we must come to realize that mistakes are not evidence of failure, but signs that we need to keep practicing. Practice makes perfect, they say.

There are many salient points about food habits that I will be taking up in this book. We will be discussing the fact that when life is not going the way we think it should, when we have an unpleasant job, an unpleasant marriage, a loveless life, we often turn to eating, and we do this as a crutch. This is not the way to live. Eating should be a happy, pleasurable process, but it shouldn't be a substitute for something that isn't going right in our life. We need to take care of problems that tend to alter our food habits, and get on with the business of life.

When we use a balanced, high-fiber food regimen to lose weight, we are giving our body the utmost support in meeting nutritional needs while taking off excess pounds. By the time you finish reading this book, you will understand why so many weight loss diets invite rebound weight gain after dieting is over, and why mine does not. You will learn how the body and mind readjust to weight changes and to changes in food intake, and how nature's reversal process will not only help you reduce but give you greater vitality and energy.

Now let me say that *I don't believe that an unnatural diet plan or reducing program will help you reach and stay at your natural weight.* The overwhelming evidence from many research studies is that 95% of those who go on crash diets regain all or more than their old weight within one year. That's nearly everyone who diets! Researchers may yet come up with an effective, relatively permanent weight control plan, but I feel we can't top nature. Our bodies and minds are made to conform to certain natural laws and principles, and it is by staying within those laws and principles that we feel and look our best. This is what I have taught for over 50 years. This is what has brought the best results for my patients.

The program presented in this book is aimed at mature adults who are willing to use will power to practice living right until they are living right and not just practicing.

One of the simplest and most effective diet procedures I know is to take a normal helping of good wholesome food at mealtime, then separate one-third to one-half of each food item off to the side of the plate and eat only the rest. This can also be varied by the amount of exercise you do.

Just as fat develops from eating more food than we expend in energy, its loss depends on eating less than we expend in energy. This is the reversal process well known to those familiar with the body's natural means of getting rid of disease. The wonderful thing about our weight-loss diet is that our body adjusts well to our program, so we don't experience the extreme sense of deprivation during the diet or the rebound weight gain afterward. I realize you can lose weight faster with drugs, extreme exercise, imbalanced diets, fasting and other available methods, but my way is one of the safest and best ways to go. I feel nature's way is best, but sometimes we need to help her out with a little common sense.

The two greatest exercises I know for reducing are shaking the head from side-to-side at food and pushing yourself away from the table before you are full.

This is the way to discover a new "you," a slimmer, healthier you. Discipline is one of the keys.

In this book, however, I have tried to make losing weight more attractive, interesting and motivating than it would be if you relied totally on self-discipline. My 30-day diet plan, near the end of the book, includes sufficient variety in foods to please almost anyone, and it is consistent in its nutritional value and calorie content with the most up-to-date, reliable research on weight reduction. I feel it is a diet plan anyone can follow.

Anyone over 40 years of age, over 10 pounds overweight or with any chronic disease should discuss this program with their doctor before trying it. Conditions such as diabetes, hypoglycemia and heart disease can be greatly aggravated by a reducing diet.

WE ARE WHAT WE DIGEST

Many times I have said *It is not what we eat that counts but what we digest.* If the digestion is poor, we are not getting all of the good from our foods, no matter how careful we are about selecting and preparing the most nourishing possible foods. We may have to take digestive supplements as found in health food stores to aid digestion. Poor digestion may be a factor in weight problems and a good digestant can be of help.

How we conduct ourselves at the table has an effect on the digestion. In past years, participants in the Olympic Games were not allowed by their coaches to discuss anything of a negative or controversial nature at the table. Why? Because digestion is impaired by such conversation, and performance is affected adversely. The table is no place for accusation, argument, gossip, bad news or the disciplining of children. Leave work problems at work; don't bring them to the dinner table. Talk should be light, uplifting, humorous and inspiring.

Champion athletes tend to avoid fried foods, cold foods, greasy foods, and having liquids with meals. This is part of their program for staying as fit as possible, and we should follow their example. One recent study showed that Americans eat twice as much fat as they should. *The average person's food habits in the U.S. are faulty to the extreme. We need to change.*

WALKING AND SWIMMING ARE HEALTHY AND THINNING

President Harry S. Truman set a wonderful exercise example for the nation by walking to work at the White House every day. And, when I say walking, I mean vigorous walking, swinging the arms and taking long, fast strides. This is what we have to do to exercise the heart, move the blood, tone the muscles and burn away the fat. Swimming is just as good as walking and much better for those who have back problems. We have to burn off calories, besides not eating them, to make a change. Half an hour of vigorous exercise raises the metabolic rate for nearly 15 hours afterward, burning calories the whole time. Exercise brings faster results in any reducing program.

Any exercise is good if it isn't too strenuous for your age, sex and physical condition. To get the best results, however, you must exercise regularly at least five days a week.

NEED HELP? BE GOOD TO YOURSELF!

How do you respond when someone gives you a compliment? Most of us like compliments from others, but many people don't know how to be good to themselves. It is not difficult for an overweight person to develop low self esteem and to begin thinking negatively about himself. This brings no benefit to anyone.

To begin a healthy lifestyle, start by looking on the bright side. Accept your body. Like yourself. You are unique, and there is no one else quite like you on the whole planet. There are things only you can do. If you have to have a regular program to break out of a low self-esteem pattern, then get up 10 minutes earlier every morning to change it. When people feel neglected, hungry for approval and affection, lacking the love they feel they need, they often turn to calories, especially sweets. This can be changed.

Don't be afraid to say silly things like, *I appreciate myself. I accept my body and am learning to love it. I am thankful for my gifts and talents.* When you pass a mirror or stand in front of one, smile and practice liking yourself. Say, *I have the power to decide how I am going to live my life.* Be sure to say it out loud.

Sometimes people think of snacking or overeating as a way of rewarding themselves. There are many better ways you can be good to yourself besides eating. Select alternatives, such as taking a nice walk, going shopping or getting involved with a hobby.

THE WHOLISTIC VIEW

Our emphasis, in taking the wholistic approach, is not to treat the **symptom** of overweight, but to take care of the whole person on the other end of that symptom. Then the weight will generally normalize.

I don't like to bring religion into this, but I have to say that for many persons, the problem of overweight could have a spiritual basis. There are certain universal spiritual laws we should keep, such as *Love thy neighbor as thyself,* and *Forgive those who despitefully use you* to reach our fullest life potential. There are many others. Spiritual laws are not optional. They must be followed to get the best out of life. We all have our lessons to learn, and the purpose of spiritual laws is to show us what our full potentials are in life.

At the mental or psychological level, there are many reasons why people become overweight. One of my patients would overeat because he feared never getting enough. Others snacked when they were bored or depressed, and they seemed to be bored or depressed quite often. We have to honestly confront and admit to ourselves why we overeat, and in one chapter of this book, I present a list of questions to help you become more aware of why and when you overeat.

Physically, there are a variety of causes of excess weight. Glandular imbalance is one. Inherited genetic traits may influence weight. Diabetes may stimulate excess weight gain or may be a result of improper food habits. Poor diet, faulty digestion or imbalanced assimilation can cause weight gain. There are, of course, many more, but the most common cause of excess weight is habitual overeating, pure and simple, and the next cause is lack of sufficient exercise.

Losing weight is simple, but not easy. You can, however, make any weight loss program much easier to follow if you muster up will power, courage, imagination, resolve and a sincere desire to change to a way of life that is specifically suited for you. That is, coordinate all spiritual, mental and physical resources to achieve your goal of finding and keeping a healthy lifestyle. Write down weight loss goals and work for them. You will get there. You can overcome any problem in which your own choices and decisions are the key to its solution.

Most animals in their natural environments are lithe and slim with bright eyes, glossy coats, quick reflexes and strong muscles. They live very close to the vegetable kingdom in the foods they eat. Most animals stay trim on fresh fruits, vegetables, seeds, grasses and so forth. The predators eat fresh meat unadulterated by hormones or antibiotics, and they eat the organ meats first, which are rich in vitamins, minerals and high-quality protein. Animals in nature eat ***WHOLE, PURE, NATURAL FOODS,*** getting plenty of exercise as they search for their food.

Man dries, cans and preserves his fruits in sugar and chemical additives, refines his sugar and flour, and packages many refined foods so they are high in calories and low in food values. Processing and refining white flour removes all bran and fiber and 22 vitamins and minerals. Many prepared foods today have more calories than the body was designed to use. If we stay more with the ***WHOLE, PURE, NATURAL FOODS,*** we will be getting more nutritional value and fewer calories.

All diets are made up of protein, carbohydrates and fats from meat, fish, poultry, dairy products, fruit, vegetables, grains, seeds, nuts and legumes. Our diet near the end of the book is especially balanced with selections of these foods in proportions recommended by the National Academy of Sciences, but conforming closely to nature's principles of whole, pure and natural. Keep in mind that a diet can have the ***proportions*** right and the ***calories*** right but can still be ***wrong*** for your body. There is a great deal of difference between a pound of sugar (1739 calories) and a pound of spinach (113 calories), nutritionally speaking. Spinach is high in food value; sugar is not.

In the back of this book, we present charts of approved foods as close to natural, whole and pure as possible, with the calories they represent. This will make it easier for you to stay healthy as you lose weight.

I strongly recommend that you see a doctor before going on this or any diet, to make sure that physical problems are not responsible for your overweight. I have found certain lab tests helpful in determining any special nutritional needs to be considered while you are dieting. It is useful for overweight persons to have a thyroid test, and I also recommend the SMA Panel, a complete blood count and urinalysis. This can help reveal glandular imbalance, possible anemia, mineral levels and other potential problem areas. Anemia, for example, can make weight reduction very difficult; it should be taken care of before beginning my weight reduction plan. Most deficiencies will be taken care of by the *Health and Harmony Food Regimen*.

In *Slender Me Naturally*, I am sharing the knowledge needed for you to succeed in losing weight and staying fit. These are things you need to know, and I urge you to read slowly, thoughtfully and carefully. It has taken me 50 years to find out and confirm much of the information presented here, and it will be very useful to you.

Impatience, as you will find, is one of the worst enemies of weight-loss dieting and is evidently self-defeating, while the best friend of slenderizing is a positive outlook, one of confidence and expectation.

THE WINNING ATTITUDE

I believe all you need to be able to lose the weight you want to lose is the right knowledge and the knowledge that you are doing the right thing. Part of what we teach here is how to have a winning attitude.

Through the first part of the book, you will acquire knowledge; then you will be equipped to put our *30-Day Diet Plan* to work. Go into this process knowing it is going to work for you, knowing that you will be able to shape up and have the body you want.

We are leaving the *Diet Plan* until last so you will be ready and eager to put it to work.

I realize there are some harsh facts in this book, and we need to know these things, while realizing that none of us is perfect. Learn from them, but don't be disturbed by them. Take life one step at a time.

No one ever appreciated a gift handed to him on a silver platter. Everyone appreciates a gift they earn through effort and perseverence. Perhaps the most valuable gift you will ever give yourself is a *"new You!"*

1

Are You An Obesity Statistic?

A recent survey showed that about 60% of all Americans are overweight, 30% of them falling in the category of obese. Obesity is defined as the condition of being more than 20% over the ideal body weight, based on a person's sex, age, height and build. In the *Ten State Nutrition Survey*, 25% of adult men and 42% of adult women were classified as obese. Dr. George Bray of the University of Southern California has said there are 4.2 million men and 7.9 million women more than 50 pounds overweight in the USA.

Perhaps this is not surprising in an affluent society where food is abundant and where most people can easily buy and eat as much food as they wish. But it is a problem—a major health problem—and I feel we must consider obesity as we would a disease. A dis-ease starts as a dis-harmony, an imbalance in the body, the lifestyle or both. We haven't been taught how to organize our eating program properly. Our plan, later in this book, will help you do that.

OBESITY IS RISKY TO HEALTH

According to the U.S. Senator George McGovern, *Six of the ten leading causes of death in the United States have been connected to the diet: heart disease, cancer, stroke, hypertension, diabetes, arteriosclerosis and cirrhosis of the liver. One third of the U.S. population is overweight to a degree which has been shown to diminish life expectancy. Obesity is a*

1

risk factor in many diseases such as heart disease, hypertension, diabetes, gallbladder disease and arthritis. *Substantial preliminary evidence indicates that nutritional imbalances in the diet contribute to at least 30% of cancer cases in men and 50% in women.*

The key words in the previous sentence are *nutritional imbalances.* It is not only the **quantity** of food we eat that determines whether we become overweight, but the **quality** and **variety.** Anemia, venous congestion, poor salivation and autointoxication may also contribute to obesity.

A MEAT-AND-POTATOES MENU IS NOT ENOUGH

The *U.S. Department of Agriculture* reports that the top-ranked foods in the country are **red meats**, followed by **bread, milk** and **potatoes**. The following survey shows an interesting food pattern in the U.S., one that helps account for the rising obesity and chronic disease statistics. My comments follow the item in parentheses. Of those surveyed:

75% eat potatoes at least 1 in every 3 days *(Potatoes and meat are a poor age-old combination of which we eat too much.)*

61% eat red meat every day.

58% eat bread every day *(People eat too much bread, squeezing out fruits and vegetables they should have.)*

55% drink milk every day *(Doctors make a living on people who drink too much milk and eat too much wheat.)*

51% eat lettuce 1 in 3 days *(No food value in iceberg lettuce.)*

50% drink coffee 1 in 3 days *(Not a natural food has side effects from caffeine.)*

50% drink soft drinks 1 in 3 days *(Side effects from caffeine, saccharine, sugars we don't need. Also, sugar is high in calories.)*

43% eat chicken 1 in 3 days *(Are there other protein options?)*

38% drink tea 1 in 3 days *(Drink only herb teas.)*

36% drink orange juice 1 in 3 days *(Not enough variety in juices.)*

28% eat tomatoes 1 in 3 days *(Good.)*

17% eat bananas 1 in 3 days *(Good.)*

16% eat apples 1 in 3 days *(Good.)*

15% eat frankfurters 1 in 3 days *(High in chemical additives.)*

10% eat cabbage 1 in 3 days *(Good.)*

10% eat hamburgers 1 in 3 days *(What else do they eat with them? Cola drinks and French fries!)*

8% drink beer 1 in 3 days *(Builds "belly" muscles.)*

5% drink wine 1 in 3 days *(Is it necessary?)*

5% eat celery 1 in 3 days *(Good.)*

5% eat carrots 1 in 3 days *(Good.)*

We are squeezing out the amount and variety of fruits and vegetables that we should eat by concentrating too much on the foods listed here.

During a recent year, Americans reportedly spent over $130 billion on junk food. Snack foods alone, such as potato chips, pretzels and crackers brought in $20 billion. An estimated 50 billion hamburgers are consumed each year and 20 billion hotdogs, along with an average of about 400 12-ounce cans of soft drinks per person. Breakfast cereals, called *empty calories* by nutritionists, now include brands with as much sugar content as candy, according to the ***Center for Science in the Public Interest***. In a pamphlet titled *Fast Foods and the American Diet*, researchers reported that foods obtained from fast food restaurants were high in salt and calories. A Gallup survey in 1983 showed 2 of every 3 adults take out food from restaurants at least once a month and about 1 out of 4 at least once a week.

Snacks, fast foods and junk foods have nourishment but are usually heavy in calories and are not nutritionally balanced. Whole, pure and natural foods increase the probability that a person will be able to stay near his or her ideal weight. Dr. Robert Good of the Sloan-Kettering Cancer Center has said that the person living on an average 2800-calorie diet would live longer and stay healthier if he cut his calories by 1/3 and his fat intake by 1/2.

Dr. George Briggs, Professor of Nutrition at the University of California at Berkeley, testified before the U.S. Senate Select Committee on Nutrition and Human Needs that improved nutrition might cut the nation's health bill by 1/3.

TAKE A WALK!

It is estimated that fat makes up about 40-50% of the American caloric intake, as compared with 10-15% of the average Asian diet. Complex carbohydrates (fresh fruits, vegetables, whole cereal grains, etc.) the dominant source of food energy in the U.S. in past years, declined from 43% of the average food intake in 1909 to 29% in 1978. Many people get a third of their energy from "foodless foods" that provide almost no vitamins and minerals. Refined carbohydrates especially sugar, leach B-vitamins from the body; put stress on the pancreas, adrenal glands and liver; cause putrefaction in the bowel; impede peristaltic motion; and are easily converted to fat. White sugar, white flour, white rice and products made from them are the most commonly used refined carbohydrates.

EFFECTS OF BEING OVERWEIGHT

Excess weight poses a variety of problems, physically and mentally. For one thing, carrying a load of 20, 30, 40 or more extra pounds all day requires extra energy and food intake. It's like a backpack that can't be taken off when you want to rest, which causes a continual burden on the heart. Because the extra weight stimulates extra eating, it tends to be a self-defeating, fat-sustaining process.

In a 1978 review in the **Canadian Medical Association Journal**, Dr. A. Angel discussed the various changes in the body associated with obesity. Adipose tissue, made of large round cells which store fat and cholesterol, increases in quantity, supported by collagen tissue and fed by many additionally needed blood vessels. Blood lipids are increased, especially triglycerides. Sugar and alcoholic beverages cause additional increase in triglycerides. Low density lipoproteins which carry cholesterol in the bloodstream increase, while high density lipoproteins, which tend to decrease cholesterol, diminish. Fat breaks down the "good" high-density lipoproteins that normally carry off cholesterol. Cholesterol production by the liver is increased, leading to higher risk of heart disease, while each pound of fat requires miles more of blood vessels, putting extra stress on the heart.

Facts like these, I realize, are not inspirational, and I want to remind you that *your goal of becoming the person you want to be is the inspiration that should carry you along.* Let these facts work to remind you of how worthwhile and wonderful your goal is, and how much good you will get oiut of it.

Cardiovascular System. Obesity overworks the heart, increases the chance of heart disease and high blood pressure, and dramatically increases atherosclerosis, the fatty deposit in the linings of artery walls that reduces artery diameter, restricts blood flow and can lead to heart attack or stroke.

Lymphatic System. The lymphatic system is a network of vessels throughout the body that contains 45 pints of fluid, as compared with 14 pints of blood in the circulatory system. Unlike the blood, the lymph has no "heart" to pump it through its system of vessels. Instead, the lymph is "squeezed" along by muscle contractions during the course of normal physical activity. As people become overweight, the inevitable result is less and less physical activity, less and less movement of the lymph. Since the lymph carries nutrients to the cells and waste products from them (among its other activities), the result is congestion and accumulation of catarrh, metabolic wastes and toxins, which creates a favorable environment for disease. Excess sodium intake increases the amount of water held in the lymph system, a further complication.

Pulmonary System. We find that the greater the bulk of the body, the more oxygen we need, yet the size of the adult lungs is fixed. Because the lungs can't meet the demand for increased oxygen, the cells and tissues of the body work under an oxygen deficit. Abdominal fat presses against the lungs and limits breathing, a further restriction on oxygen intake. All cells, all metabolic processes in the body require oxygen, and we find that oxygen deficiency as a result of overweight lowers the level of function of every organ, gland and tissue in the body. Obesity is a serious complication in cases of asthma.

Gastrointestinal System. The fatty tissue throughout the body of obese persons tends to make the bowel flaccid, leading to prolapsus of the transverse colon, balloon conditions, bowel pockets, underactivity and constipation in many cases. Displacement of the stomach into the chest cavity is more common in overweight individuals. An overworked, underactive bowel allows more toxic materials to enter the bloodstream, from which they are deposited in the fatty tissues and inherently weak organs and tissues of the body.

Skeletal System—Joints. Overweight persons experience greater wear and tear on their joints, especially in cases of arthritis or spinal problems such as slipped or ruptured disks. The discomfort and irritation of painful joints further reduces physical activity in overweight persons, favoring more weight gain and a general increase in associated health problems.

Liver and Gallbladder. Because of lowered physical activity, bowel underactivity and lymphatic congestion, the liver must work hard to deal with detoxification, reducing its capacity to perform its many other tasks. This may be one reason why more gallbladder disease is found in overweight persons. One study showed that 88% of 215 people operated on for gallstones were overweight.

Overweight persons tend to be dissatisfied with their appearance and with the increased physical limitations that come with excess weight. Often there is guilt associated with eating patterns and sensitivity toward comments by others about weight or appearance. They may become depressed or develop low self-esteem.

TELEVISION AND OVEREATING

Television advertising, in my opinion, contributes greatly to guilt associated with being overweight. Beautiful young men and women with slender, well-proportioned bodies are shown using or promoting products, pretending to have a wonderful time. The impression is given that you have to be young and slender to have a good time.

On the other hand, TV ads present food after food—candy bars, snack foods, cereals, cakes, cookies, donuts, steaks, waffles, fast foods and so forth, and some of these look so wonderful they almost appear better than the real thing. So, we are constantly bombarded with TV ads that encourage us to buy and eat the things that make us fat, while being told we have to look young and slim to enjoy life.

INFLUENCES ON OUR EATING HABITS

Dr. Beverly Winicoff of the Rockefeller Foundation has pointed out that our eating habits are influenced not only by our upbringing but also by what is available at the supermarket, school cafeteria, restaurants, airports and places of work. She points out, *We put candy machines in our schools, serve high-fat lunches to our children and place cigarette machines in our work places. The American marketplace provides easy access to sweet soft drinks, high-sugar cereals, candies, cakes and high-fat beef, and more difficult access to foods likely to improve national nutritional health.* Dr. Winicoff stated that people seemed to believe doctors could cure the various diseases that come from poor eating habits. *There is, in reality,* she said, *very little that medical science can do to return a patient to normal physiological function.* We might add that even hospitals have candy and cigarette machines.

OTHER REASONS WHY PEOPLE ARE OVERWEIGHT

Cultural patterns may induce people to be overweight in several ways. In some countries or regions, excess weight is considered a sign of wealth or high social position. In others, the lifestyle may be slow and easy, allowing more food to be turned into fat. Some cultures keep their women relatively confined to the homes of parents, husbands or other relatives, which encourages overweight from inactivity and boredom. In a few Middle East countries, overweight women are considered more beautiful. Japanese sumo wrestlers deliberately get as fat as they can and as strong as possible, because both weight and strength are important factors in their sport.

Climate and altitude, terrain and level of technology, influence the weight. There are people who gain weight rapidly in wet tropical climates but lose it in a dry or temperate climate. There are people who gain weight at sea level but lose it in the mountains. Hot weather helps some keep slender, while cold weather favors others.

Genetic factors influence weight. I don't exactly like comparing people to horses, but it is useful to realize that some people are built large like draft horses while others are more streamlined like racehorses. There is a "right" weight for each, but it is not the same, even for the same height. Good curves, by their nature, are looked upon as beautiful, whether the frame is small or large.

When you stop and think about it, there is no such thing as an "average" person. We are all unique. But there is a natural "normal" weight for each of us.

WATER RETENTION AND OBESITY

It has been said that there are some people who can look at a glass of water and gain half a pound on the spot. This is an exaggeration, of course, but there are a considerable number of people who tend to retain water in their tissues, and this is a problem for them. Dr. V. G. Rocine classified such people as hydripheric types or lymph types.

Many women are familiar with a tendency to bloating that comes usually before menstruation each month. In such cases, endocrine hormone shifts are causing water retention. We also find that endocrine imbalance can be an ongoing problem in some persons, without regard to the menstrual cycle, holding excess water in the body.

Another cause of water retention is imbalance in the sodium-potassium ratio in the body. Excessive table salt intake can trigger this imbalance, and the solution is simply to cut back on salt intake and to eat more foods that are high in potassium.

Weight-loss gimmicks that promise rapid results often rely on water loss, but they do not burn off enough fat to do any good so they are useless.

An estimated 25 million Americans take diuretic pills to control high blood pressure and many of them have found they can "cheat" a little by using their pills for weight reduction. Diuretics work by causing the excretion of more water, and some have discovered they can lose 6-8 pounds in 2 days. This is extremely dangerous. Potassium, which is very important in the body, is also excreted. Some potassium-depleted patients have had to go on kidney dialysis machines because of kidney damage. Potassium is needed by the muscles, especially the heart muscle, so that loss of this mineral can produce muscle weakness and eventual heart damage. Excess use of diuretics can cause death.

There are safer ways to lose water. Cut back on salt, as previously suggested. KB-11 and cleaver tea are herbal diuretics, much safer than diuretic pills. Vitamin B-6 can be used, up to a gram a day, with relative safety. Some who have taken several grams of B-6 per day have experienced problems with the nerves in their wrists. It is possible to overdose with some vitamins, so it is best to investigate what the maximum safe level is.

FAD DIETS ARE NOT THE ANSWER

Every year, millions of Americans go through the ritual of starving their bodies down to some desired weight, only to gain it all back again in the next few months. They take special diet pills, powdered mixes, eat certain fruits and stay away from fattening foods—for a while. Then they fall back into their old living habits again. Newspaper columnist Ralph Moyed estimated that he has lost 485 pounds since 1977 on various diets and visits to "fat farms" as he calls them, and gained nearly all of it back. Many people are familiar with the yo-yo process of gaining and losing weight, over and over.

At any given time, approximately 40 million Americans are on diets. In his book **Rating the Diets**, Theodore Berland mentions more than 75 diets. In 1941, we had the grapefruit diet. Then it was the steak and tomato diet, the egg and orange juice diet, the drinking man's diet, the macrobiotic diet and others. In 1977, a liquid diet protein drink boomed into a popular fad, and 17 persons died from trying to live on the diet drink alone. Current diet powders, designed to be mixed with liquids, have more nutrients, but 6 persons using one of them have died. An estimated 5 million Americans have tried the new diet powders.

The danger of the new powders is that many provide only 330 to 500 calories a day, which is basically a starvation or fasting diet. Muscle wasting, water loss, nutritional imbalance, endocrine system imbalance, fatigue and other serious health problems can occur as a result of following such a diet. No diet under 1000 calories per day for women or 1500 calories per day for men should be attempted without a doctor's supervision or advice.

We find that the average person is simply not well enough informed about food, nutrition and the workings of the body to safely conduct a fast or an extreme low calorie program of weight loss. Losing weight too rapidly may damage the organs and glands and nearly always creates a rebound effect. Over 95% of those who use fad diets to reduce their weight gain it back within a year, according to Dr. George L. Blackburn of Harvard Medical School.

If fad diets, diet powders and diet pills were the solution to the problem of obesity, it would have been solved long ago. We need to realize, however, that it is not the diet program that loses or gains weight, it is the person. It is necessary to pay attention to and take care of the person at the other end of the weight problem to achieve lasting, permanent results.

The ritual of periodic, repeated dieting to take care of periodic, repeated weight gain is only a symptom of a more basic underlying problem. And, let me say, I don't believe the problem is the same for everyone. We are all unique individuals, different in the ways we think and feel, different in the ways our bodies respond to foods, different in the ways we handle the stresses and experiences of life. We don't have the same size or strength in the functional ability of our organs. There is a solution to undesirable weight gain, and it can only be found by seeking a right way of living and sticking to it.

NATURE SHOWS THE WAY

For over 50 years, I have worked with patients, using natural methods to bring people back to health. Many of those years were spent in sanitarium settings in which I lived and worked with my patients day after day, week after week, trying to help each one find a permanent solution to the ailment or condition they were trying to get rid of. I discovered that nature cures, but sometimes she needs an opportunity.

Chronic disease builds up in the body in most cases from faulty eating and living habits over a period of years. In this sense, obesity can many times be classified as a chronic disease. Fat develops slowly, just like many chronic diseases, when our metabolism has been thrown off balance. The best way to take care of it is to look to nature for the answer, just as I have done in taking care of other health problems.

The problem with modern civilization and a high standard of living is that man looks away from the great encyclopedia of nature and bases his lifestyle on what contemporary technology has to offer. Too many people take on a self-indulgent philosophy, get into the fast lane of life and proceed to eat, drink, work, smoke and worry themselves into disease. The way back to a permanent state of health lies in reversing the process by which the disease was acquired, not in some temporary treatment of symptoms. Treating symptoms does not remove the cause.

THE REVERSAL PROCESS

The first step on the reversal path is to stop doing those things which contribute to the problem or disease. The second step involves cleansing the body of debris and toxic waste that are contributing to the problem.

Cleansing may be helped by diet, properly supervised fasting, bowel management techniques, exercise or hard physical work, selected herbs and other supplements and reducing the stress of life problems. When the body tissue has been adequately cleansed, the next step is to go on a food regimen based on whole, pure and natural foods. Tissue can only be rejuvenated or rebuilt with nutrients from foods. My *30-Day Diet Plan* will help cleanse the body as well as reduce the weight. Reducing the amount of fatty tissue on the body is essentially a reversal process, with many side benefits.

There were no can openers in the Garden of Eden. Adam and Eve had no frying pan, and they were not tempted by hundreds of TV ads to eat sugary or salty or fat-fried foods devoid of most nutritional value. They did not plug up their bowels with processed fiberless foods, nor did they go out to fast-food restaurants twice a week. Their foods were natural, pure and whole, and they had no diseases and no excess fat. Fad diets would not exist if we had not departed so far from the food principles of the Garden of Eden.

Most diets aim at getting rid of the symptom—fat. My diet plan is different. My approach is to help you understand why you are overweight, then assist you in discovering a better, more natural and appropriate food regimen and lifestyle, a way of life that will bring you sufficient peace and satisfaction that you can leave diets behind and simply live a healthy way of life.

When we find the higher path in life, will power increases to a level where we take control over what we eat, think, feel and do with ourselves. As our life improves, so does our will power. We need will power. We need to know we are doing the right thing. Psychologists say that the strength of our will power is related to general muscle tone. My program is designed for adults who are willing to use their will power to do the right thing in their lives.

Reaching a weight that is right for you and staying there depends upon your willingness to recognize and leave behind those aspects of your lifestyle that cause overweight. The reward is great—good health is a door through which we must walk to find the best things in life.

I believe there is a natural weight for everybody. It may not be exactly what the statistical charts say we should weigh, but it is the proper weight where each individual is disease-free and feels at his or her best.

2

Why
You
Gain Weight

There are many reasons why people put on extra "padding," some psychological and some physical. However, we find that too often experts attempt to separate the mental realm from the physical realm, leaving us with two disconnected sets of explanations for problems such as obesity, and this can be misleading. Everything that happens to the body or inside the body affects the mind; every thought, emotion, perception, attitude or belief affects the body.

Disease can cause obesity, and obesity can cause disease. We find that studies have shown the mortality rate from diabetes in men over 45 increases 10 times in those who are 26% overweight as compared to normal-weight men. Obesity has been associated with diabetes as both a possible cause and an effect, even though the direct cause is pancreas malfunction. When the blood sugar is abnormal, food cravings are abnormal, and the reverse is also true. Scientists don't know the ultimate cause of diabetes.

Anemia, endocrine problems, venous congestion, lymphatic congestion and inadequate salivation may all contribute to obesity. Children overfed as infants may develop more fat cells than others, which can cause lifelong problems with weight control.

Overeating has many psychological factors involving self-image, the emotions, boredom, stress response and personality. The psychological and physical aspects of obesity do not exist separately or independently from one another, so we will look at them together.

WHAT DETERMINES HOW WE FEEL ABOUT OUR WEIGHT?

According to Susan C. Wooley, co-director of the Eating Disorders Clinic at the University of Cincinnati Medical Center, the current obsession with thinness is producing serious problems in today's women. She feels that today's generation of young women is the first to grow up watching their mothers, *the first generation of weight watchers, despairing over their thighs.* In a survey, only 13% of the young women participating believed their mothers liked their own bodies. Unhappy with themselves, the majority of the mothers tended to be more critical of their daughters.

I have treated five cases of anorexia in the past few years, and, believe me, many women are having a very difficult time putting food and life-style patterns into a right perspective. I taught my patients that proper eating was to be appreciated as a means of letting the best in life flow through us.

In some countries of the Middle East today, most notably Turkey, men consider plump women more attractive. Some years ago, the film **Mondo Cane** pictured an African tribal monarch with a considerable number of wives, all hugely obese. Obese wives were not only considered beautiful in that African culture, but were status symbols as well. It took a fair amount of wealth to keep a wife that well fed.

The slender feminine ideal today in the United States is just the opposite. It is almost impossible to achieve in the context of the average homelife or job. Models and actresses seen in films, magazines and on TV are paid extremely high wages compared to the average woman, and it is as much part of their job to be thin as it is to act or to model. They say a woman at her normal ideal weight appears fat on TV. Almost any woman in this country could stay thin if she were paid a thousand dollars a week or so for her trouble. Yet, only two generations ago, some men preferred women who were "pleasingly plump." This is something to stop and think about.

We find that the basic problems of those who have anorexia nervosa and bulimia are centered around a fixation on slenderness, a fear of being fat and an addiction to dieting. Dr. John Kilbourne, a university lecturer and authority on advertising, states: *"Ads are a very powerful educational force. It's difficult not to be influenced by the constant bombardment."* He notes that ads tend to make women feel guilty about

13

being overweight. In fact, diet and weight loss products are marketed by making women feel insecure about their bodies, since they see only thin women in all the ads. Basically, this is a form of psychological manipulation, and we should not be deceived by it.

The same media pressure is exerted toward men, but not to the same degree of success, perhaps because men are not as sensitive to the emotional undercurrents used in ads as women are.

Still, there is definitely something very wrong in a society in which women and men are influenced to feel guilty and unhappy about their bodies. There is something very wrong when 20% of all teenage girls have used vomiting to control their weight, as reported by Susan Wooley of the University of Cincinnati. Actress Jane Fonda spent *23 years of agony* as a bulimic, stuffing herself with food then vomiting 15 or 20 times a day. When we find millions of women using fast weight loss programs to the point of triggering natural body defenses and later bringing out a compulsive urge to gorge on food, we need to realize we are not doing the right thing.

A young woman in her 20s weighing 86 pounds came to my office at the Ranch with anorexia. For 7 years, her eating was influenced mostly by mental attitude—avoiding certain foods, choosing others, trying various diets, until her system was so imbalanced that she became seriously underweight. We put her on a harmony way of living at the Ranch and in a few months, her weight was up to 116 pounds. She followed our basic **Health and Harmony Food Regimen**, substituting vegetarian proteins for the fish, poultry, lamb and occasional lean beef allowed. When I asked her what had contributed most to overcoming her condition, she said, *You've done more toward changing my **attitude** toward food than anything else.* I feel that professional counseling is a must for any anorexia or bulimia problem.

Wrong eating habits can have a powerful effect on the nervous system, the glandular system or both, and the mind can become seriously affected. Starvation diets ultimately damage the nerves and force the glandular system and body to adjust to a lower metabolic rate. Fatigue and depression set in all too easily, along with irritability and sudden mood shifts. Psychological problems become intermingled with physical problems, and the solution to these problems will never be found until we discover that nature has something very important to teach us. We need to get away from extremes and look to nature to find out a right way to live.

14

When we eat right, get adequate rest, exercise, fresh air, sunshine and so forth, our bodies will adjust to a weight matched to a natural state of high-level well-being. You can feel wonderful. You can enjoy your body and experience the best health you've ever had. *But you must be willing to work for it!*

INHERITANCE AND INHERENT WEAKNESSES

Some people gain weight easier than others, and I believe much of this could be inherited. All doctors recognize that some people are born with weak lungs, weak kidneys, liver defects and so on. I call organs and tissues that do not function normally "inherent weaknesses," and all of us have at least a few of them. Some have many.

When we are born, we are 1/3 our father, 1/3 our mother and 1/3 ourselves. We can have a normal body even though we may have inherent weaknesses brought down from the father, mother or farther back on the family tree. We may have inherited a tendency to gain weight or we may become overweight from poor food habits traditionally used in the family. Studies have shown that obese children are 3 times as likely to become obese adults, when food habits are harder to correct. However, we have dominion over our bodies, and most inherent weaknesses can be compensated for.

An extreme genetic tendency to gain weight in my opinion, could take five to eight generations to overcome by following right living and eating methods in each generation.

We need to recognize that there are consequences when we have inherent weaknesses. The person with a pancreas weakness can't tolerate sugar the way other people can. The person with an underactive bowel can't take care of white flour products or fiberless foods the way other people can. In other words, we have to take special care of our inherent weaknesses to keep the weaker organs and tissues from breaking down and becoming vulnerable to disease or influencing our weight.

A tendency to gain weight easily may be due to a variety of inherited conditions. Because there are so many glands, nerves and organs involved in appetite, digestion, assimilation and use of nutrients, inherent weakness in one or more of them can make fatty tissue production a potential problem. In most cases, as I have mentioned, we can compensate for inherent weaknesses by proper eating, exercise and a proper mental attitude.

Among the glands and organs that have to do with fat metabolism are the hypothalamus, pituitary gland, thyroid gland, pancreas, adrenals, sex glands, liver, gallbladder and small intestine. If inherent weaknesses are found in any of these glands and organs we may have problems with weight control.

Some persons metabolize their foods faster. Some digest foods more efficiently, perhaps because of an abundance of digestive juices. Some have better mental attitudes toward food, health and themselves.

Genetic defects, as found in some glands causing a lack of certain enzymes, can also affect fat metabolism.

HOW THE GLANDS AFFECT WEIGHT GAIN

One of the undesirable side effects of low calorie fad diets under 1000 calories a day is the "starvation" response by the brain. When weight is lost too rapidly, the thyroid gland slows down to adjust the metabolism to the lower food intake, so fewer fat calories are burned. Meanwhile, the appetite center in the hypothalamus turns on the "hunger switch." As normal eating habits are later restored, a higher percentage of the food is turned to fat because the body energy requirements have been lowered, and the "hunger switch" in the brain stays on until all the old lost weight has been "found" again. These diets are self defeating because of the way our brain works.

The pituitary is the master gland of the endocrine gland system, and doctors have found that tumors of the pituitary and other types of pituitary malfunction can contribute to obesity. The pituitary is connected to the hypothalamus of the brain (where the appetite center is) by both nerves and blood vessels. Neurohormones secreted by the hypothalamus influence the secretions of the pituitary, which, in turn, affect the various other glands. Keep in mind that the appetite center is associated with blood levels of various nutrients, and I believe this also has an influence on the pituitary.

Why are these things important? Because imbalance of the sex hormone estrogen can trigger obesity, and the adrenal hormone aldosterone controls water retention in the body. The amount of salt we use in foods, among other factors, affects the aldosterone level in the body. Fasting diets, by dramatically altering nutrient levels and balances

16

in the body, can disrupt the glandular system, leading to abnormal weight gain later. The short-term success in weight loss leads to long-term failure. We must know about these things to avoid the pitfalls that catch so many dieters.

Dr. Weston Price believed that a diet high in refined carbohydrates, particularly white sugar, threw the endocrine system out of balance. An imbalanced endocrine system can open the door to many disorders, but one of the most common is obesity.

A malfunctioning pituitary gland, an underactive thyroid, adrenals that cannot control the sodium-potassium balance in the blood and sex glands with an imbalanced estrogen production can all contribute to obesity.

Emotional upset or strain can break down the thyroid gland to the point where it becomes hypoactive, leading to unwanted weight gain. Sexual disappointment or disturbance can lead to sex gland imbalance, resulting in excess weight gain.

The glands need lecithin, protein and cholesterol to function properly. Cholesterol, seldom deficient in the body, needs to be balanced by lecithin. Those with high blood cholesterol, generally speaking, would do better to take more lecithin than to cut back on cholesterol in foods, although I do not approve of fatty meats or fat-fried foods for other reasons than cholesterol content. We find that the thyroid needs adequate iodine to function properly and we can get iodine from halibut, sea bass, tuna, salmon, red snapper, rock cod, fish roe, kelp products, dulse, onions and various fruits and vegetables grown near the sea coast.

MENOPAUSAL WEIGHT GAIN

Weight gain after menopause is often a very frustrating experience for a woman, because the changes in body chemistry are so complex it is difficult to know what to do. I believe the best way to approach change of life weight problems is to make sure the body has all the minerals needed to come to its new equilibrium as gracefully as possible.

Menopause weight gain is usually due to endocrine system adjustments as discussed in the previous section. Sometimes the herbs black cohosh and licorice are very helpful to women going through the change of life, and men will find that ginseng and fo ti tieng will help balance the glands.

Adequate exercise is needed to keep the body toned, the blood and lymph moving and the bowel functioning properly. Exercise is even more vital in the later years than for the young, but heavy exercise should be avoided.

THE MENTAL SIDE OF THE WEIGHT PROBLEM

It is fascinating to consider that the appetite center is in the hypothalamus, which has been called the psychosomatic center of the brain. Nerves from every tissue and organ in the body converge on this brain center, as well as nerves from the emotional and thinking areas of the brain. Here is where thoughts and emotions affect the blood chemistry and the automatic functions of the body, down to the cell level, and, on the other hand, the blood chemistry and metabolic functions affect the thoughts and emotions. The way we think and feel can help us become fat or thin.

I had a patient once who failed to lose weight despite being on an excellent reducing regimen I had given him. When I questioned him about it, he admitted he was eating a whole broiled chicken every night, because he had a deep-seated fear of not getting his "fair" share of food. He overate because of a fear of not getting enough.

The housekeeper of the famous violinist Fritz Kreisler could tell by the kind of music he was practicing what kind of meals to serve him. If he was playing difficult classical music, he was exacting in his meals. But, if he was playing waltzes or other light music, he wasn't so strict in what he wanted to eat. Music affects mood, mood affects mind, and mind is then affected in its food choices.

There are people who feel they have to "Keep up with the Joneses" in the expense, quantity and refinement of the foods they eat. If you serve food you think your guests will like, you have to eat it too. Most of us have had the experience of going out with people, then ordering what they order (or ordering what we think will impress them) whether it is good for us or not. Similarly, we have all been guests at the homes of others where we had to eat what they served. You can see how the mind affects how we handle ourselves in such cases. We can usually eat more of the vegetables and leave the refined starches alone. We have to be selective to eat properly, regardless of circumstances.

There are many times, I think, that instead of eating we should get busy at some job or hobby or **take a walk**—anything to take the place of the craving for food. Many times these cravings are abnormal and don't represent a real need for food. Some people are like Pavlov's dog—whenever the bell rings they are ready to eat. Others are stuck in schedules. They always have breakfast at 7am, lunch at noon and supper at 6pm. Their minds are trained to think "food" at certain times whether the stomach is hungry or not. I feel it is not a good idea to eat unless we are hungry.

We find that many people allow food to draw them around like a bull with a ring in its nose. When it is time to eat, we eat, not because we have to but because it is a habit. Eating or drinking should not be a hobby, avocation or something we always think of when we have time or money on our hands. Many people can't get their minds off food, which can cause them a lot of trouble.

Some people don't eat, they "breathe" their food in. They take in everything they can. They work on their plate like they are vacuuming a rug. Once we had a group at the Ranch who complained that they didn't get enough to eat when we served the food on plates, so I put the food out in buffet style and let them help themselves. One man filled his plate four times at one meal, and I told him, "You are going to kill yourself eating all that food." He said, "I'm paying for it, so I'm going to get all I can." This is a bad attitude, and sometimes our attitude is what kills us. We find out that we are capable of eating enough to fill a much larger dress or suit than we should fill, and this is where we need to apply common sense and discipline.

Some people overeat when they are bored, depressed, unhappy or feel unloved. Others lose their appetite when they fall in love, lose their job, have an argument with their spouse or suffer an emotional shock of any kind.

One survey we have mentioned showed that 87% of the mothers of teenage girls probably do not like their bodies. What does a thought like that do to the appetite center? When we look at the extreme effects of emotion and thought in anorexia and bulimia cases, it is overwhelmingly evident that what goes on in our minds has much to do with how we eat, what we eat, how much and how often we eat, and how our bodies process what goes into them.

Cigarettes, amphetamines and diet pills all suppress the appetite center by drugging it, but as soon as the drug is taken away, more weight is put on than before. Suppression never really works and is almost always counterproductive in the long run. Unnatural forms of weight loss probably all have undesirable side effects and long term effects.

PERCEPTION AND OVEREATING

We know the brain monitors glucose levels in the blood and is capable of triggering hunger in the appetite center when glucose falls too low. But we can also become stimulated to hunger, even when the body has adequate nutrients circulating, by the sight or smell of food. So, we know the visual and smell centers of the brain are connected to the appetite center.

Unfortunately, foods that are bad for us can be very appealing, and a bad diet can cause obesity.

BRAIN CONTROL OF WEIGHT AND APPETITE

In recent years, some researchers have come to believe that some part of the brain "decides" on how much fat our bodies need, and that we eat until we have it. I believe this is nonsense, because if it were true, many people in other countries besides ours who have access to plenty of food would be "overweight," and we find that obesity is more of a problem in the United States than in most other places.

What I believe is that the body may get used to the amount of fat it contains, and some center in the brain considers this fat "normal" after a period of months or years. After all, fat is not dead matter. It has blood vessels and nerves running through it. It affects the center of balance, the blood chemistry, the amount of work the heart does and many other functions.

If the brain considers a certain amount of fat natural to the body, it will be alarmed at rapid weight loss, assuming it indicates potential imbalance of body chemistry and function. This is why the metabolism drops, to conserve energy and to keep functions going at a lower level of energy use and food intake. The brain's appetite center is very patient and stores up a long-term hunger which is geared for new weight gain once the diet is ended. *All permanent weight loss programs must take this effect into account to be successful.* There is at least one way to overcome this problem, which we will take up later.

Scientists once thought that overweight people were psychologically different from people who were not overweight. More recent research indicates that psychological differences come after the weight gain and because of it, not before.

THE DIGESTIVE PROCESS AND OBESITY

Most overweight problems boil down to overeating, and even what we don't eat. When we eat more of the right foods, we eat less of the wrong foods. When we neglect to eat the right foods we develop chemical deficiencies in the body. It's as simple as that. And, even knowing how the digestive process works can help us learn to keep the food intake under control.

When we eat, digestion begins in the mouth as salivary enzymes begin changing starches into sugars. In the stomach, the food is churned up, broken down into fine particles and mixed with hydrochloric acid and enzymes. Protein is broken down into molecules called polypeptides. The liquefied stomach contents are squirted into the beginning of the small intestine. Pancreatic enzymes plus bile from the liver are secreted into the small intestine. The pancreas completes digestion of starches, and assists in the breakdown of proteins and fats. Fats are emulsified by the bile and made ready for absorption. Tiny, finger-like projections along the small intestine called villi then begin picking up the digested, broken-down microscopic food particles and absorbing them into the bloodstream.

All food-carrying blood vessels from the small intestine empty into a single large blood vessel which goes to the liver. The liver, one of the largest and most important organs in the body, processes proteins, fats and starches. Components of proteins called amino acids are sent out for cell building and repair, glucose is sent to cells for energy and fats are sent out bearing the fat-soluble vitamins, such as A and E. The liver stores extra glucose as glycogen, but when its storage requirements are met, the excess glucose is made into fatty acids. Excess proteins may be broken down into waste acids such as urea and excreted through the kidneys, but they may also be converted to blood sugars or fat. A common misconception is that a high protein, low carbohydrate, low fat diet is an effective reducing diet. Not necessarily. We may have a digestive

21

problem. Your doctor may recommend digest aids and Pancreatin with meals. As I said before, any food can add extra weight under certain circumstances. We need to think in terms of a balanced food regimen.

OBESITY AND THE BOWEL

The importance of bowel regularity and colon hygiene have been all but forgotten by the great majority of doctors in our time. A sluggish colon, constipation and bowel irregularity have two consequences that favor obesity in a certain type of people. The longer waste material remains in the bowel, the more fats and cholesterol are absorbed into the bloodstream. The same is true of toxic waste products. The latter circulate in the bloodstream, and some appear to get past the liver, the great detoxifier of the body, to deposit in inherently weak glands and organs. Toxic settlements lower the metabolism of tissue where they settle, which in some cases allows greater buildup of fat.

SUMMARY—WHY YOU GAIN WEIGHT

The following list summarizes the causes currently known at the root of obesity and unwanted weight gain.

1. OVEREATING
When we eat more calories than we use up in daily activities, we gain weight—mostly fat.

2. GENETIC INHERITANCE
Our inherent weaknesses can predispose us to obesity. We may lack enzymes needed to break down fat and expel it.

3. ENDOCRINE IMBALANCE
Imbalance in the endocrine glandular system can cause obesity, particularly the pituitary, thyroid, pancreas, adrenals and sex glands.

4. POOR DIET

A poor diet can cause obesity directly or through endocrine imbalance.

5. MENOPAUSE

This is basically a glandular system adjustment.

6. RAPID WEIGHT-LOSS DIETS

These usually encourage even more rapid weight gain afterward.

7. PSYCHOLOGICAL PROBLEMS

Many people tend to snack and overeat when they are bored, depressed, unhappy and feel unloved. Insecurity feelings may contribute to overeating.

8. BRAIN CENTERS

Brain centers tend to protect the status quo, even when the status quo is unwanted fat. The basic problem is still overeating.

9. DIGESTIVE PROBLEMS

Liver or pancreas malfunctions may have an effect on weight gain, but may be caused by poor eating habits in the first place. A toxic bowel, a constipated bowel, encourages reabsorption of cholesterol from bile and toxic deposits in tissues, which lower metabolism and encourage weight gain.

10. DEFICIENCIES

What we *don't eat* as well as what we *do eat* can cause nutrient deficiencies in the body that encourage weight gain. Lack of exercise contributes to extra pounds.

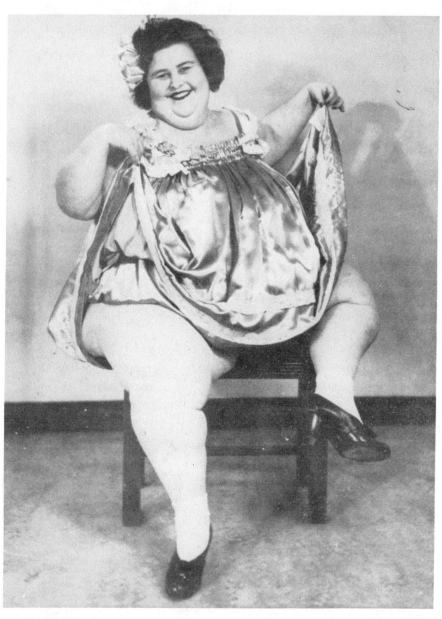

Dolly Dimple was a circus fat lady who weighed 555 lb but realized that something could be done and should be done to come down to a more normal healthy weight. Over several years, using a doctor-supervised balanced reducing diet like those in Ch 10, she lost weight very gradually and nicely until she weighed 118 lb.

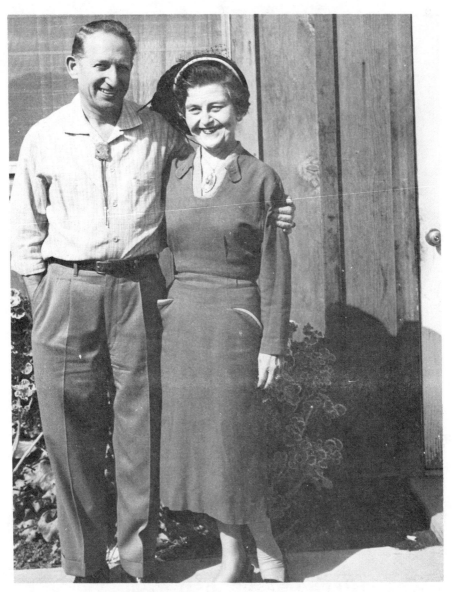

During this "reversal process," as we call it in the natural healing arts, she had a healing crisis which brought back an extreme fever and other symptoms she had at age 5. Sometimes it is events in the early years that trigger the health problems of later years. Everyone should know about the reversal process and the healing crisis which comes with this natural program. Dolly Dimple was an extreme case, and I want to say that my average overweight patient is generally only 10 to 50 pounds overweight.

3

How Much Should You Weigh?

When the Creator designed the human body, I don't believe He intended to have it come out assembly-line style, with all women destined to weigh 123 pounds and all men 165 pounds. There are individual differences that give us a certain amount of leeway in these matters, and it is best to make our peace with the fact that we are not all going to look like movie stars or models.

We need to learn to be the best we can be, then accept what we are and be glad about it. In the previous chapter, we saw how most standards of beauty—whether fat, medium or thin—are determined culturally. There is no inherent reason why we should let other people decide how much we should weigh or how we should look. I believe nature knows best, and if we look to her for our answers, we will not be disappointed. If we try to be something we are not, we are asking for trouble.

No one can say with absolute assurance what you should weigh. But they can get close. Scientific research, population studies, statistics and insurance company studies have contributed greatly to our understanding of how much a person of a certain height and build should weigh to have the healthiest possible life. So, we know closely, if not exactly, about how much you should weigh.

THE NOTION OF "IDEAL WEIGHT"

I believe there is an ideal weight for everyone, a weight naturally suited to us by virtue of our height, skeletal framework, metabolism and inheritance. The problem is, *no formula discovered by science can calculate this.*

Some researchers say if you are 20% above or below your "ideal" weight and you feel well and fit, don't worry about it. We can't force everyone into the same mold. I believe it could be possible that our weight should vary, at least slightly, with occupation. That is, if the same person had a job doing active physical labor for three years, then transferred to a desk job, I would expect some readjustment of the body in terms of metabolism, enzyme activity, nutrient processing and weight.

When I traveled around the world, searching for the secrets of longevity by talking to the oldest men and women in each country, many of them over 120 years old, I found that most weighed the same as they had from age 20 to 30. These people were in excellent health. Other researchers say a slight weight gain (up to 20%) is to be expected as we grow older.

Still another research project indicates that if people stayed slightly under their ideal weights, they might live up to 30% longer. The study was done with laboratory rats who were consistently underfed, compared to a control group of rats who were allowed to eat all they wanted. When I visited the Hunza Valley some years ago, many of the old men and women, still healthy although well over 100 years old, were as slim as they had been in their 20s. They seemed to eat less at meals than the average person in the U.S.

Not all ideas of what makes a healthy or beautiful body center around ideal weight. Adolf Just believed that body symmetry was more important. He measured Grecian curves and came up with a unique standard for what constitutes a healthy body, based on looks instead of weight.

Let's realize that the ultimate goal must be a healthy body, a body free of disease with plenty of vitality and high-level well-being. If you try to sustain a weight that is too slim for your constitution, you will not feel your best physically or mentally.

There are different charts for ideal weight, and the one we use is among the best.

Because of body chemistry and hormonal differences, women carry more adipose tissue on their bodies than men, which accounts for the soft, graceful curvature of their bodies.

Children, from infancy through the teens, may go through changes in body fat related to changing metabolism and body chemistry, but I want to make clear that obesity in children is just as hard on them, with almost the same risks and dangers, as for adults. The reasons children become overweight are about the same as for adults. In overeating, the only difference is that the parent, not the child, bears responsibility.

Now, look up the ideal weight for your height, build and sex on the weight chart below. Consider whether it could reasonably be judged too high or too low for you. (It may be helpful to discuss this with your spouse.)

Decide on a weight goal that you can put your heart into achieving, and write it down on 3 x 5 cards or pieces of paper. Then put one on the wall in the bathroom, one in the kitchen, one in every room where you will see it relatively often and at strategic times of day. These constant reminders of your goal will help you stick to it.

WOMEN				MEN			
	Weight (without clothing)				Weight (without clothing)		
Height (without shoes)	BODY FRAME			Height (without shoes)	BODY FRAME		
	Sml	Med	Lge		Sml	Med	Lge
5 feet	100	109	118	5 ft 3 in.	118	129	141
5 ft 1 in.	104	112	121	5 ft 4 in.	122	133	145
5 ft 2 in.	107	115	125	5 ft 5 in.	126	137	149
5 ft 3 in.	110	118	128	5 ft 6 in.	130	142	155
5 ft 4 in.	113	122	132	5 ft 7 in.	134	147	161
5 ft 5 in.	116	125	135	5 ft 8 in.	139	151	166
5 ft 6 in.	120	129	139	5 ft 9 in.	143	155	170
5 ft 7 in.	123	132	142	5 ft 10 in.	147	159	174
5 ft 8 in.	126	136	146	5 ft 11 in.	150	163	178
5 ft 9 in.	130	140	151	6 feet	154	167	183
5 ft 10 in.	133	144	156	6 ft. 1 in.	158	171	188
5 ft 11 in.	137	148	161	6 ft. 2 in.	162	175	192
6 feet	141	152	166	6 ft 3 in.	165	178	195

The Right Way
to Count Calories

Almost everyone has some idea of what calories are from watching television advertisements of diet soft drinks. Too many calories make us fat, and fewer calories will keep us slimmer. This is approximately true, but it is certainly not sufficient to help us know what a healthy food regimen is. We need to understand that *all* foods have calories, but *only whole, pure, natural foods* build health.

A *calorie*, as defined in nutritional studies, *is the amount of heat energy required to raise the temperature of a kilogram of water one degree Celsius.* The calories in most common foods have been determined by laboratory tests, and the calories of work energy it takes to perform different kinds of activities and jobs have also been measured. It is not difficult to compute how many calories we need per day to get through the various things we do, and that determines how many calories we need in our food intake each day.

If we take in more calories than we use, the excess turns into fat. When we realize that it takes 3,500 calories to make a pound of fat, we can see how one soft drink a day (which comes to 55,000 calories a year!) can cause us to put on nearly 16 pounds of weight annually. This is why we have to watch what we eat, especially when we are past the active "calorie-burning years."

In my travels around the world, I have met many old men and a few old women who were perfectly healthy while over a hundred years old. Not one of them used a high-calorie diet. Not one of them overate or used junk foods.

It isn't only the number of calories that counts, but the quality of foods we get them from. *The National Academy of Sciences* has recommended that our daily food intake average 16% protein, 20% fat and 64% carbohydrates. This is less protein and fat and more carbohydrates than the average American adult consumes, but it is basically a healthier diet. We also need a certain amount of water, vitamins and minerals each day.

Be careful just counting calories. All foods provide calories, but not all are **NATURAL, PURE AND WHOLE** as they should be.

My *Health and Harmony Food Regimen*, described in a later chapter, will make clear what I consider quality foods. I just want to say I don't believe in junk foods, fried foods, refined carbohydrates (such as white sugar and white flour) or packaged foods, which are usually dead foods preserved by chemicals. None of these kinds of foods are natural to our bodies, and I believe they are often fattening and always harmful to our health, no matter how many or few calories they have. Abnormal foods build abnormal bodies.

People have come to consider anything they put in their mouths as food, but that is not true. When we stop and think about it, only those substances which promote life and health in us qualify as foods. Real food is essential for the growth, life, repair and replacement of cells and tissues, and it gives us the energy we need to function in our daily lives. Most kinds of food are composed of seven basic elements—water, protein, carbohydrates, fats, fiber, minerals and vitamins.

Processed "foods" often lack sufficient vitamins and minerals to properly process and use the protein, carbohydrates and fat they contain. That's why I call them "foodless foods," and others refer to them as "empty calories."

The best foods for us are foods that are whole, natural, pure and fresh. I believe in plenty of fresh fruits and vegetables eaten mostly raw. I believe in using fresh meat whenever possible, preferably fish (the kind with white meat, fins and scales), chicken, turkey, lamb and, occasionally, lean beef. I do not believe in eating fatty meats, pork or manufactured meat products such as hotdogs. Meat should be broiled, roasted or baked, and vegetables should be cooked in waterless stainless steel cookware or steamed to preserve the enzymes, vitamins and minerals as much as possible. Potatoes, yams and sweet potatoes, may be baked in their skins (and eat them sparingly). *Potatoes should be eaten with skins, to provide minerals, vitamins and fiber.*

THE BASICS OF WEIGHT LOSS

If it takes 3,500 calories of food to build a pound of fat, it will take 3,500 calories of energy to burn up that same pound. The basic strategy in weight loss is to use up more calories than you eat each day, which means you must exercise more, eat less or do both. Eating less has faster results, and I would add that if we reduce wisely and eat quality food (although less of it) we will stay healthy and well during and after the diet.

Because it takes more calories simply to maintain an overweight body than one at the ideal weight, we can expect to encounter an energy lag at some point as we shift from a higher to lower weight. The less junk food, coffee, alcohol and other valueless food and drink you take in, the more available energy you will have, but any energy drop you experience is only temporary.

As explained in a previous chapter, the brain doesn't know you are dieting but sees the lower food intake as starvation, which brings an inherent survival mechanism into play. The thyroid slows down energy use throughout the body, and metabolism slows down to balance with the lower food use. This is what brings in the energy lag. At the same time, the brain stores in its memory the fact that the body is losing weight, which will be regained later. This weight "deficit" is then activated when the person goes off the diet. All this is done below the level of consciousness, *with all fast weight-loss diets.*

Another thing going on is that all the enzymes in the body which were busy building and maintaining fat are still there, but many of them are now "unemployed," so to speak. These "unemployed" enzymes are thought to play a role in both the relentless hunger response after the diet and the rebound weight-gain effect.

Keep in mind, we are talking about *rapid weight loss*, which I do not endorse or approve unless done under a doctor's supervision. Rapid weight loss can cause all sorts of problems for the body and mind, and such diets are usually counterproductive. Research shows that 95% of those who lose weight on crash diets gain it back within a year.

The correct way to lose weight is to take it off slowly enough that the brain, nerves and endocrine glands can adjust to the new weight without triggering the starvation response and bringing in the rebound weight-gain effect. Impatience is our worst enemy in dieting. We want to see the bathroom scale show results—fast. It can be done fast, as we know from experience. But it is time to face the facts and recognize that rapid weight loss with very low calorie diets simply doesn't work. The fat comes back.

MORE THAN WILL POWER IS NEEDED

We find that we can't override the innate wisdom and survival instinct of the body on sheer will power alone, because brain mechanisms are involved that have nothing to do with will power.

Some years ago, a clever research scientist devised a diet experiment with a group of volunteers to see if automatic brain regulating mechanisms could be fooled. The volunteers were given access to automatic pushbutton dispensers of a liquid diet drink and were told they could drink as much as they wanted, just so they wrote down the amount in a record book. The liquid was tasty, nutritionally balanced and fortified with vitamins and minerals. It had a carefully measured number of calories per glass.

After several days when the researcher knew the amount of the liquid each person drank per day (and the number of calories), he cut the number of calories in half without telling the people. That is, he diluted the drink in such a way that the taste, consistency and appearance remained the same. Only the calories were changed, which the subjects had no way of knowing.

The first day of the change, most people drank their usual amount. The second day, all increased their intake. Within several days, all subjects had doubled their liquid diet consumption, giving them the same number of calories they had before. The brain is not fooled by the sight, smell and taste of food into taking too few calories.

Related experiments were done with rats at the Massachusetts Institute of Technology, and researchers found carbohydrate intake was regulated by a brain chemical. Eating carbohydrates increased the amount of the neurotransmitter serotonin, which decreased the hunger signal from the brain when the rats had eaten enough. The serotonin apparently builds up in the brain and shuts off the "switch" in the appetite center when a sufficient number of carbohydrate calories have been taken. Researchers varied the taste of the rats' food, but they still ate the same daily total amount of carbohydrates. They varied the percentage of carbohydrate and the rats still ate the same amount. Regulatory control over carbohydrate intake had to be in the brain, since taste, smell, sight and varied percentages of carbohydrate in the feed showed no influence over the rats' total carbohydrate consumption.

Researchers then investigated dieters using high protein, low carbohydrate reducing diets. After dieters came off their diets, researchers found out it took twice as much carbohydrate as before the diet to build up the same serotonin level. In other words, the high protein, low carbohydrate diet had somehow messed up the carbohydrate-regulating system in the body, and those who were trying to eat normal meals again were not feeling satisfied until they had eaten twice as much starchy foods and sugary foods per day as they had before they started dieting. This is the rebound effect. This is why many people regain all of or more than the weight lost while dieting.

One major difference between the food habits of people and rats is that people are more influenced by the sensory appeal of foods. It is easier for people to overeat than rats. How food looks, smells, tastes, sounds and feels in the mouth can influence people to overeat. Sweet foods or drinks and salty foods are easy for many to overconsume, and for some, they seem to be addictive.

In another experiment, 23 overweight subjects were given a choice between protein snacks and carbohydrate snacks. Most chose carbohydrates nearly all the time, and had snack cravings at special times like midafternoon or just before bed. The problem was not will power but chemical imbalance. When these subjects were given a drug that raised serotonin levels, their snacking dropped dramatically.

I feel the eating habits of most people, especially in the overeating of protein, fatty foods and refined carbohydrates, has created abnormal conditions in the appetite center of the brain. Ordinary crash dieting simply produces further imbalances. The average fat intake per day in the U.S. is 40-50% of the daily food taken, twice as much as the amount recommended by the National Academy of Sciences. Getting back to a healthy, right way of eating is the ultimate solution to weight problems.

There is a correct way to take in fats. We can get all the fats we need when we use foods such as whole milk, eggs, avocadoes, nuts, nut butters and other natural foods. Our bodies can handle and digest fats properly when they are a natural ingredient in foods. Concentrated fats and oils are much more difficult for the body to take care of.

TAKE A WALK!

HOW WE USE UP CALORIES

During a 24-hour day, we burn up a certain number of calories which varies according to what we do. Basal metabolism, the operation of all body functions in the resting state, takes about a calorie per minute, or 480 calories during an 8-hour sleep period. In our waking hours, exercise, household tasks, driving, job activities, walking, talking and other normal aspects of life use up energy at varying rates. Calorie expenditures for a variety of activities are given in the following chart.

Surprisingly, perhaps, the major benefit of exercise is not in keeping the weight down by burning up fat, but in keeping the appetite center normalized, moving the blood and lymph, toning and firming the muscles and strengthening the heart. However, exercise does increase the metabolism for up to 15 hours, and more fat is burned off. Research has shown that a combination of exercise and balanced diet is the very best way to reduce weight and keep it off. Fast weight loss just doesn't work over the long term. Patience is a key factor. Weight loss at a rate of 1 or 2 pounds a week allows the brain and body chemistry to rebalance and readjust, without triggering the "rebound effect" of gaining back all the old pounds.

Based on average activity levels for the average American, the following calorie charts have been worked out. Keep in mind that these figures are not intended to provide more than rough guidelines.

Calorie requirements vary considerably from individual to individual, but these charts will give you some idea of how many calories you normally need to get from your food to maintain a healthy weight.

CALORIES BURNED PER HOUR FOR VARIOUS ACTIVITIES

Activity	Per Pound Ideal Weight
Awake, reclining	0.50
Bicycling	1.10
Bookbinding	1.10
Carpentry	1.56
Dancing	1.95
Dishwashing	0.93
Dressing/undressing	0.81
Driving car	0.88
Eating	0.65
Exercise, light	1.10
moderate	1.88
strenuous	2.90
very strenuous	3.90
Ironing	0.93
Knitting	0.73
Laundering	1.05
Painting	1.56
Peeling potatoes	0.75
Playing a cello	0.98
a piano	0.84
a violin	0.77
ping pong	2.50
Reading aloud	0.69
Running (5.7 mph)	3.70
Sawing wood	3.12
Sewing by hand	0.72
by machine	0.74
Singing	0.79
Sitting relaxed	0.65
Skating	2.10
Sleeping	0.43
Standing at attention	0.74
relaxed	0.69
Stone working	2.60
Sweeping	1.09
Swimming	3.25
Tailoring	0.88
Typing rapidly	0.91
Walking downstairs	2.36
slowly	1.30
moderately fast	1.95
very fast	4.22
Walking up stairs	7.18
Writing	0.69
Vacuum cleaning	1.78

HOW TO USE THIS CHART

Look at the chart on the next page and find your ideal weight. For example, if you are a 5-ft, 2-in. female with a medium body frame, your ideal weight is 115 lb (no matter what your real weight is). If you have gone out dancing for 2 hours and want to know how many calories you have used, simply multiply your ideal weight (115 lb) by 1.95, the calories per hour used up per pound of ideal weight, as shown on the Calories Burned Per Hoiur chart, then multiply again by the number of hours—2. So, we have 115 × 1.95 × 2 = 448.5 calories. If you had only danced a half hour, it would be 115× 1.95 × 0.5, or 112.1 calories.

DAILY DIETARY CALORIES NEEDED

Females				Males			
Age	Ideal Weight	Height (in.)	Calories	Age	Ideal Weight	Height (in.)	Calories
10-12	77	56	2250	10-12	77	55	2500
12-14	97	61	2300	12-14	95	59	2700
14-16	114	62	2400	14-18	130	67	3000
16-18	119	63	2300	18-22	147	69	2800
18-22	128	64	2000	22-35	154	69	2800
22-35	128	64	2000	35-55	154	68	2600
35-55	128	63	1850	55-75+	154	67	2400
55-75+	128	62	1700				

FOODLESS FOODS TO STAY AWAY FROM

Your ultimate goal should be to get away from diets, to find a healthy way of living where you won't need to diet. Plan on developing healthy eating habits so your weight will stay where it is supposed to be. My diet plan is designed to help you do that, but it will not work unless you resolve to stay away from foods which are worthless or harmful to your health.

The following list of undesirable foods is not intended to be complete, but from it you can gain a clear understanding of what types of foods to leave alone. In general, all packaged foods and all foods containing chemical additives should not be eaten, because processing has robbed them of valuable nutrients and because any added chemicals are a potential danger to health, no matter what the food industry says about their supposed safety. The best philosophy of eating is to stay with natural, whole, pure foods as closely as possible, most of them raw. Some vegetables and all grains and meats need to be cooked. We will get into this more later. Many frozen fruits and vegetables are all right, but some frozen products are processed or adulterated with chemicals, so read the labels.

Most people will stray from a good diet now and then, and it is not what we do once in a while that harms our bodies, so I do not take an extreme position on such things. But, you will find that as you eat more whole, pure and natural foods, you will lose the desire for many unnatural foods. Sweets will not have the same appeal. Fat-fried foods often become repulsive. Heavily salted snack foods will lose charm. While you are making the transition to a better diet, however, it is best not to have junk food in the house. Resist temptation by avoiding it altogether.

FOODS TO AVOID

White sugar and products
   containing white sugar
White flour and products
   containing white flour
White rice
Soft drinks (including diet drinks)
Chocolate
Beer
Ale
Hard liquor
Dried fruit, sulphured
Canned food containing
   chemical additives
Beef jerky
Smoked meat, fowl or fish
Fatty meats
Dry packaged breakfast
   cereals (except muesli
   and whole grains)
Chili
Coffee
Crackers (except sesame, Ak-Mak, etc.)
Any food substitute
Highly seasoned foods
Fruit, unripe
Sweetened or artificial fruit drinks
Ice cream
Macaroni
Marshmallows
Peanut butter

Pies
Potatoes, peeled, mashed or fried
Saccharin
Spaghetti
Sweet desserts
Tea (not herbal)
Packaged luncheon meats
Cakes, cookies, donuts and pastries
Candy
Catsup
Chips (potato, corn, etc.)
Cornstarch
Condensed milk
Egg substitutes
Fried foods
French rolls and bread
Fudge
Hominy
Hot cakes
Lard
Malted milk
Noodles
Pickles
Pork and beans
Pretzels
Puddings, packaged
Salt
Syrup
Tapioca

The right way to count calories is to start with foods that count for health. Our digestive system, appetite control center and body chemistry are designed to work properly with foods that are natural, whole and pure. Adulterated foods, unripe foods, processed foods, man-made foods and wrongly cooked foods tend to cause disturbances that eventually develop into serious health problems, vitamin and mineral deficiencies and toxic settlements in the body. They also contribute generously to obesity.

One of the greatest aids I know in losing excess weight is raw foods. Have plenty of salads, using a variety of ingredients. Use fresh fruits as desserts or between meal snacks. Have carrots, celery, radishes, sliced cucumbers, tomatoes, bell pepper slices or other raw vegetables you like, in the refrigerator all the time, to have with meals or between meals. There are few calories but many valuable nutrients in raw vegetables. Fruits have more vitamins but are higher in calories, so I advise only two a day as compared with six vegetables. I advise dropping wheat, milk and sugar from your food regimen completely because most people have had so much of them that they have developed an abnormal body.

5

*Think Right
To Keep Fit*

One of the great paradoxes in life is that we must think right to have good health and we must have good health to think right. Thinking right, thinking vigorously, and the joyful feelings that come out of a mind that works effectively, help balance the glandular system, especially the thyroid. While you are slimming down to a healthy weight, keeping in mind that you intend to stay there, resolve to change habits of thinking that may contribute to unwanted weight gain.

Here are some typical patterns of thinking that contribute to excess weight:

"I don't want to see these leftovers go to waste." (The economy excuse.)

"I've been so good today—got the kids off to school, finished the laundry and ironing, did the shopping—so I deserve a nice big piece of German chocolate cake." (The reward excuse.)

"I'm so mad (or frustrated or disappointed, etc.) at my wife (husband), I'm just going to have a big helping of cherry pie ala mode." (The revenge excuse.)

"Let's get out the cokes, chips and popcorn—our favorite TV show is on." (The TV excuse.)

"It's 3 o'clock—time for my tea, toast and jam." (The time excuse.)

"Aunt Helen's coming over, so we're going to have her favorite dessert—angel food cake and strawberry ice cream." (The visitor excuse.)

"The Hansens are such big eaters, we'd better have steak, potatoes, vegetables, salad and dessert when they come to dinner." (The keep-up-with-the-Hansen's excuse.)

"Surely, a few hors d'oeuvres won't hurt." (The little-bit-is-okay excuse.)

There are other habits of thinking that get us in trouble; we will discuss more of them later. The nice thing is, when we see our habits down on paper like this, we can laugh about them, then make a decision to change. While will power isn't everything, without it, weight control is impossible, so let's realize a fact of life from the start: *EVERYBODY HAS WILL POWER.* All you have to do is learn to develop what you have and use it.

A DIET QUIZ FOR YOU

To assist in identifying areas of your life and thinking that may be obstacles to weight control for you, answer the following questions and think about your responses. There is no answer list to check your results; the object is simply to help you understand more about your food priorities and habits.

1. In comparison with other pleasures and satisfactions in your life, rate eating on a scale of 1 to 10.

2. In terms of your various priorities right now, rate being at the "right weight" on a scale of 1 to 10.

3. Can you think of more than two reasons why you would like to be slim?

4. Are you impatient to lose weight?

5. Do you consider dieting difficult or unpleasant?

6. Are you resentful toward yourself for being overweight?

7. Have you dieted before? How many times?

8. Do you look forward to getting off your diet so you can eat certain foods you shouldn't have again?

9. Do you tend to eat more when you are fatigued?

10. How close to bedtime do you eat dinner? Is dinner your largest meal of the day?

11. Do you think other people find dieting easier than you?

12. Do you have difficulty saying, "No, thank you," when someone offers you a drink or snack that you know is fattening?

13. Do you believe thin people can eat all they want?

14. Are there foods you would go out in the evening to buy if you found you were out of them?

15. Are there friends of yours with whom your main pastime is eating?

16. If you have dieted before, was your main reason to appear more attractive, then return to your old lifestyle?

17. Before you read this book, were you aware that being overweight increased your chances of acquiring one or more of several diseases?

18. In terms of your other goals and priorities, rate being in good health on a scale of 1 to 10.

19. Is it hard for you to visualize yourself as a slim person?

20. If you have dieted before, did you continue to look into other reducing diets, diet pills, weight-loss methods and so on?

21. Do you think about or fantasize about certain foods?

22. Can you think of one, two or three foods that may be key foods in getting or keeping you overweight?

23. Do you have a hard time stopping once you've started eating them?

24. Do you tend to snack when you are bored or depressed?

25. Do you snack at certain times of day? In certain rooms of the house or certain restaurants or coffee shops?

26. When you realize you have eaten more than you should during a single meal, do you continue to eat?

27. If you overeat at a couple of meals, do you give up on your diet and drop it?

28. Do you believe staying at the right weight would change your life in ways you would enjoy?

29. On a scale of 1 to 10, rate how difficult you believe staying at your right weight would be.

30. Have you ever considered that changing aspects of your lifestyle could make staying slim much easier?

Try to spend at least ten minutes reviewing and thinking about your answers. One of the keys to weight loss and better health is understanding your own life patterns, motivation and personality.

MIND OVER "PLATTER"

Like it or not, our mind is married to our body, "for better or for worse." And, it can be for better, as we learn to think our way to right living.

We have previously mentioned that the appetite center is located in a uniquely important part of the brain—the hypothalamus—which brings many mental faculties to bear on our eating habits. Both the thinking brain (cerebral cortex) and the emotional brain (limbic system) are linked to the hypothalamus—and, therefore, the appetite center—by important nerve channels. The hypothalamus also controls and monitors our endocrine glands, which dramatically affect how we think, feel and behave. It does this via the pituitary gland, the "master gland" of the body.

We find that every thought, every feeling, affects every one of the billions of cells our body is made of. They do this by their effects on the nervous system and the glands. We must realize, if we are overweight, that our thoughts and emotions have contributed to the development of the problem in the first place and help maintain it in the second place—no matter what other causes there may be. A healthy, positive attitude and peace of mind toward **both our present physical appearance and our future slender goal set us free to succeed** in our goal.

There are a lot of people who gain weight when they stop smoking. Now, if a person has the willpower to stop smoking, he could use that willpower to stop eating so much and could fortify himself with a more balanced diet, foods that will not cause fat. Many of us eat from our feelings and not from our actual need for food. We find out when we feel good that we eat entirely differently than when we are morbid or depressed.

Overeating in a land of plenty such as the U.S. is not a subject so profound that we need to keep analyzing the situation. What is often abnormal, however, is what people do and think once the evidence of overeating is obvious to the individual and everyone else. Excess weight is a symptom that something is wrong with that person's body and lifestyle, just as symptoms of other chronic diseases are nature's way of telling us something is wrong. The right thing to do at that point is to remedy the situation, learn the lesson and correct the problem. And, the simple lesson in most cases of obesity is to eat less until our weight normalizes, then stick to a balanced food plan such as my Health and Harmony Food Regimen.

CARE ENOUGH TO SAY "NO"

The first step in overcoming an undisciplined eating habit is to learn to say "no." One young lady allowed herself to get fat because she couldn't say "no" to aggressive men interested only in sex; getting fat solved that problem but made her unattractive, which she didn't like. When she learned to say "no" to men, she felt comfortable slimming down again.

It is not wrong to enjoy food. But, it is not right to abuse our bodies through overeating and this problem is not so difficult to correct. We have to put "mind over platter."

As we have said previously, some people eat when they are bored, depressed, nervous, anxious or unloved. There are effective ways to deal with these problems, but eating is not one of them. When we believe that eating helps us feel better, then get disgusted when we see the fat that results, we are internalizing a mental conflict that invites a host of problems.

Discipline is not a gift or talent, it is a learned behavior which starts with an attitude of willingness to overcome. We can start to develop it by saying "no" in the case of small things in life, such as sleeping an extra 10 minutes in the morning, a second cup of coffee with breakfast, an invitation to gossip or downgrade someone. Once you have experienced the power and authority of saying "no" to little things, go on to bigger and better things. Say "no" to second helpings. Say "no" to gravies. Say "no" to watching TV in the afternoon when you could be taking a walk. Say "yes" to things you know are good for your body, mind and spirit. Discipline has its "yes" side, too.

Insecurity, low self-esteem, suppressed aggression, anger, resentment, bitternes and other emotional disharmonies can manifest in overeating, possibly by causing imbalance in the appetite center as well as through purely psychological means such as substitutional or compensatory behaviors.

People who aren't satisfied with their love and sex life often turn to food. It is very important to have the sex life right so that substitutionary behaviors don't bring in some kind of imbalance. Foods, especially sweets, are among the most satisfying activities to most people, but we can't trade one thing for another and expect the body to stay in balance. The correction of lifestyle imbalance should be made in the original part of the lifestyle that was disturbed.

THINKING AND SPEAKING THINNESS

Some years ago, a major East Coast university conducted a survey of the words used by people in ordinary daily conversations and found that a high percentage of the average conversation was negative or critical. This, I believe affects the body adversely.

Do you speak negatively about yourself? Do you think and speak critically of your own body, habits, characteristics, behavior or abilities? Previously, we said that higher brain functions such as thought were connected to the part of the brain that houses the appetite center. I believe the appetite center is affected by our speech and thoughts, and if we throw it out of balance, our eating habits can become abnormal and possibly the way our body digests, assimilates and uses nutrients as well.

Specifically, I want you to stop thinking and saying things like: "I'm too fat," "I have a terrible weight problem," "I don't like the way I look," "All this flab looks terrible," "Everybody notices how fat I am," and "I feel miserable because of my weight." For each of these kinds of things you find yourself thinking or saying, substitute statements that indicate work or improvement, such as "I feel better now that I'm doing something about my weight problem," or "I'm becoming slimmer every day."

Some years back, one of the popular weight control programs came up with the slogan, "Think thin." This is a wonderful idea. Think of yourself as thin. Think of your appetite as under control. Think of yourself as a person of authority who can say "no" to fattening food and drink, a person who can walk past a refrigerator without a second glance.

Ladies, imagine yourself in a lovely new dress, one or two sizes smaller. Men, imagine yourself in a good-looking suit with a leaner wasteline by 4 or more inches. Picture these in your mind frequently to help build motivation. Some persons have actually gone to a department store and bought smaller size dresses or suits in advance, then hung them in the closet to look at every day until they fit. And, of course, they do fit. The body follows the mind, the imagination, the will.

Can you see what we are getting at in this chapter? Can you see how what you think and say can be a wonderful, constructive help in shedding unwanted weight and staying as fit as you like? Learn to use language as a tool for accomplishing goals, such as losing a specific number of pounds and following a better lifestyle. Think in terms of success, of winning, of anticipating good results.

LOVE AS A REDUCING AID

As I have said before, many people who feel unloved overeat. Now, this is a serious problem, because the person who feels unloved really doesn't care if he or she is overweight, and the heart of the problem here is not gluttony but loneliness. The problem is lack of a feeling of self-worth, of being lovable.

I have seen cases where feeling unloved produced glandular imbalance. The thyroid is the "emotional gland," very susceptible to emotional influence, and we find that an underactive thyroid can lead to unwanted weight gain even without overeating. We also find a loss of willpower, a loss of discipline when a person feels unloved. This is something we have to take care of. We need to be around people who love us for our own good. We have to leave old things behind and take on a new and better way of life.

In many cases of overweight problems, I have sensed that the excess weight was not going to leave until the person was willing to let go of something. It seemed as though the fat was being held in place by an unwillingness to change, to let go of the old and take on a new life. We can't hold on to grievances, bitter memories and old problems without consequences to our body and our health.

WHAT ARE YOU CARRYING?

Is there a spiritual problem? Let go of it and make your peace with the Almighty. Are you resisting, resenting and holding onto bad memories? Forgive the people involved. Do you feel unloved? Find someone who needs a friend and love them. You have to let go of the old and take on the new. Life is a flowing process; nothing is meant to stand still. Are you around mean, spiteful people? Find people who like you and leave the others behind.

The Good Book says, "Love your neighbor as yourself," My mother once taught me, "We have to love other people for our *own* good." Think about that. I don't say it's easy, but it's true. We can't love our neighbor unless we love ourselves, but maybe the key to loving ourselves is to show love to others first. Kindness is precious, and people appreciate it very much. Like love, it is one of those things that blesses those who give as well as those who receive. The best way of breaking out of the feeling of being unloved is to start doing something for other people. Love flowing through you is healing. You will soon feel loved.

Don't wait around for someone to bring love to you first. You take the first step.

Love is a healer, because it releases those things in the mind that have grown stagnant and toxic. We can't love and feel bad at the same time. We can't love and hold onto bitter memories at the same time. Love truimphs over all obstacles. Love is always just right. And, in this sense, I believe love can be a reducing aid.

MOTIVATION AND REDUCING

Obviously you wouldn't be reading this book if you didn't have some degree of motivation to reduce your weight. But, we find it is often helpful to examine our motivations, to check their consistency with our various goals in life. The basic question, once again, is "Why do you want to lose weight?"

The reason we bring up the question is because many people *do not* want to lose weight. They want to appear attractive or athletic. They want to radiate sex appeal. They want to impress the boss, to increase chances of promotion. Or, they want to lose enough weight so they won't gain again when they get back to a normal food regimen. None of these people really want to lose weight. They want something else, but they have to lose weight to get it.

Now, I don't think there is anything wrong with these things, but is there any reason you can't raise your sights a little and say, "I want to lose weight because I want to be as healthy as possible and to feel as wonderful as possible?" Stop and think about it. When you take the path to better health all these other benefits come with it. You get a lot more than you get from a reducing diet, and it stays with you.

As I have said before, I believe the reason why 95% of all those who use reducing diets gain back the weight they lost within a year is because they go back to their old lifestyle.

What's wrong with the old lifestyle? Too much to cover here, but I want to point out a few reasons why so many people's lifestyles are unhealthy in the U.S. Poor food choices, lack of exercise, too little fresh air and sunshine, staying up too late, excessive use of drugs and alcohol, chronic marriage problems, too much rushing around, pollution, traffic, excessive noise, not enough sleep, not enough exposure to beauty, poor recreation choices and other processes that contribute more to dis-ease that to health.

What sense does it make to lose weight, then go back to a way of life dominated by other unhealthy factors? Why settle for one bite when you can have the whole apple?

Recheck your motivation: What do you really want out of life? How does good health fit in that context? What is being slimmer and feeling better going to do for you?

POSITIVE THOUGHTS FOR SUCCESSFUL REDUCING

Here are some mental exercises to do along with your diet, once you begin the program. Some call these "affirmations," others call them "auto-suggestions" or "meditations."

Sit in a comfortable chair in a quiet room where you will not be disturbed for 10 to 15 minutes. Do three of the following exercises each day; if you learn them by heart and do them from memory, so much the better. Say such one alternately aloud and silently to yourself at least 6 times.

1. LOVE

I allow love to flow into and flow out of myself, carrying away every obstacle to being a fully loving and lovable person. I will be loving toward others and toward myself, allowing my body to become healthier, stronger and slimmer, day by day.

2. AUTHORITY

I have complete authority over everything I take in at the spiritual, mental and physical level. I choose to think positive thoughts and select the right foods to make my mind clear and to help my body reach its natural weight. I can say "no" to any fattening food and "yes" to any food that is right for my body. I am in charge of choosing the times and places I will eat. I have authority over myself.

3. ENJOYMENT

I enjoy my life right now, delighting in the foods I eat, glad that I am not eating foods that put on weight, glad that I am losing weight each day. I enjoy the feeling of my body as I become more fit and slimmer, and I am thankful that changes are being made for the better in my body and mind.

4. LETTING GO OF THE OLD

I choose to let go of the old and become a new person. I choose to release any old memory that hinders my progress toward reaching my natural, healthy weight. I choose to release any old habit that has contributed t my weight problem in the past. The old has passed out of my life, and I welcome the new.

5. THANKFULNESS

I am thankful for each new day, thankful for the many wonderful things in my life and thankful for friends and loved ones. I am thankful for my health and for my peace of mind. I am thankful that my mind molds to a new way when I put the right thoughts in it. I am thankful that every day, in every way, I am succeeding in reaching my weight goal.

6. SELF-DISCIPLINE

I am completely in charge of my body and its needs, and I realize my body follows the leading of my mind. I have complete confidence that by means of correct self-discipline, my body will mold to a better, healthier, slimmer way of life. Because self-discipline is a form of love, a way of taking responsibility for my own looks, actions and health, I gladly open myself to receive the many blessings I expect from it—self-confidence, self-respect, self-control, peace of mind and greater enjoyment of life.

7. SERENITY

My nerves are strong and calm, stronger and calmer, stronger and calmer than ever before. I feel in harmony with myself, with the universe and with everything around me. I am rich with inner powers that give me harmony, security and serenity, that give me the ability to comfortably, easily and gracefully lose weight. Nothing and nobody can bring me out of unity with the Higher Powers that protect me, and I am rich with inner powers that give me harmony, security and serenity, that give me the abililty to comfortably, easily and gracefully lose weight. Nothing and nobody can bring me out of unity with the Higher Powers that protect me and make me invincible, invulnerable, unshakable.

8. VITALITY

I feel full of health and the joy of living. There is sunshine in my soul today. The clouds have rolled away, and I feel confident, reassured and ever so contented. I feel young, ever so young. Every day in every way I feel my normal weight developing and a return of more vitality. As each pound of fat melts away, I grow more energetic, more filled with vitality. I use this vitality to burn up calories. I feel like a new and powerful personality, able to overcome any obstacle with the greatest of ease. I feel wonderful—simply marvelous.

9. SLENDERNESS

Every day in every way I am growing more fit and slim. Every day in every way I am feeling better and better. Every day in every way I am growing closer to my ideal weight to the weight natural to my body. I love my body. I am at peace with myself and I know I am on the right path.

FINAL SUGGESTIONS

Don't talk a lot about your diet, but on every appropriate occasion, simply tell friends and others, "I feel wonderful! I am making changes for the better all the time."

When you find yourself thinking or daydreaming about food, change your thoughts or dreams to a beautiful natural scene such as a mountain lake or stream, or to an activity you enjoy such as roller skating, doing crossword puzzles, hiking, bird watching, going to an art gallery or whatever else you like.

Two of the greatest obstacles to success in weight loss and weight management are excuses and blaming others. When you can let go of these things and begin to take responsibility for your own life, important and wonderful changes will begin to take place. I can't tell you how valuable it is to be responsible for your own life.

One of the greatest encouragements toward succeeding in your weight-loss goal is to put a picture on the wall showing your ideal shape. This inspires the conscious mind and provides a non-verbal incentive for the unconscious mind.

6

Exercise Keeps Us Trim

Exercise isn't the easiest way to turn a person on, especially if he is busy. Busy people seem to put exercises aside, hoping that they will be able to keep the nice lithe figure that came as a free gift with youth. But, there comes a time, either in middle age or if we've been eating too much and sitting around too often, when we suddenly realize we have developed bulges in the wrong places. We develop padding over our thighs, rear end and stomach that is really difficult to get off. Seldom is anyone overjoyed at this discovery.

Of course, prevention of excess weight is best, because losing weight is very difficult to do. I think people develop self-defeating philosophies about prevention. *Why should I try to prevent something I don't have?* they ask. Weight goes on easily—and very subversively—over a long period of time. We don't notice the little quarter inch bulge that appeared at first, but six months later, it's up to a half an inch and six months more it's up to an inch. Then our best friend says something like, "Aren't you putting on a little weight?" Your belt doesn't take the same notch it used to, or your pants don't fit the same, and we have to let them out or get new ones. Of course, this book wasn't written for those who do not need to reduce, but I think it would be well if we realized some of the principles laid down in this book are for keeping us at a proper weight.

Music is a great stimulant in getting us to exercise. It virtually leads us into movement, creating such enjoyment that it takes the work out of exercise, or seems to, anyway. Be sure to try exercising to music.

To get the most from exercise, we should do it daily. Anyone who exercises three times a week will get good results from it. Those who exercise five days a week will get three times as much good out of exercising only two days more. We have presented here many more exercises than you can do, so you can select the ones that are right for your particular program and so you can change to get more variety when you are tired of one set of exercises.

A good exercise program circulates the blood into the fat tissues to dissolve it and to bring it back into the blood to be broken down and eliminated.

When we stop and think about it, the more weight we gain, the less physical activity and exercise we tend to do. We can turn that statement around, and it is just as true. The less physical activity and exercise we tend to do, the more weight we gain. It's as simple as that.

AVERAGE WEIGHT GAIN

The average American gains a pound a year after age 25, according to Dr. Jack Wilmore, physical education expert at the University of Arizona.

Exercise alone, as we have said before, is not the best way to lose weight. For example, running a mile at a pretty good clip will only burn up 120 calories, less than an ounce of fat. This can be somewhat discouraging, unless we add up all the benefits of exercise.

First, however, no one who is over 40 years old or over 10 pounds overweight should begin an exercise program without consulting a doctor. Similarly, if you have a heart condition, ulcers or any other serious physical problem, you should see a doctor about what exercises you can do. **You should also tell the doctor about the diet plan you are on when you ask his advice concerning exercise.**

It is not our purpose here to present a universal exercise plan, since exercise needs vary according to age, sex, state of health and amount of excess weight. What I want to do is show you what the benefits of exercise are, and how they fit into the kind of natural lifestyle where we look and feel our best. **The human body is designed by nature to work best when we get adequate exercise and rest. Every organ responds to exercise and proper nutrition.**

What most people don't understand is that the whole body is affected by obesity (and by weight loss). Exercise is one of the necessary ingredients for everyone's health, not just overweight people, but it is nice to know that a physically fit body burns fat calories faster, easier and more safely than a soft, flabby body. Permanent weight control, based on a right way of living, must include exercise.

Possibly the most interesting fact about exercise is that 20 to 30 minutes of vigorous activity once each day causes the basal metabolism to rise and stay up (above normal) for nearly 15 hours after exercising! This means your body is burning up calories faster than usual as you go through your normal day's work and activity, or even as you sleep. This is a bonus in speeding up weight loss.

Secondly, exercise tones the bowel and promotes regularity, which assists in weight loss. Studies have shown that the longer wastes remain in the bowel, the more cholesterol is absorbed back into the body. **Where is this extra cholesterol stored? Mostly in fat cells.**

Thirdly, we need to exercise to move the blood and lymph, stimulating good blood circulation to the brain to ensure this vital organ gets all the nutrients it needs, and moving the lymph along to get rid of bacteria, foreign matter and wastes. The blood and lymph carry off the breakdown products of fat catabolism, assisting in the weight loss process. But, we must realize the lymph system has no "heart" to act as a pump as the blood circulatory system does; **muscle movement is the only thing that moves lymph.** So, exercise is vital to the lymph circulation and in getting enough blood to the brain. The latter is particularly important, because without a sufficient blood supply, the brain would become deficient in needed nutrients and would gradually lose its efficiency in running the heart, lungs, and kidneys, liver and so on, as well as in regulating the weight.

The heart muscle is strengthened by exercise. This is important because each pound of fat, so it is said, has several miles of blood vessels and capillaries running through it, which create an extra burden on the heart. Strengthening the heart helps compensate for the stress placed on it by obesity, even as excess weight is being burned away.

The aerobic aspect of exercise promotes efficient oxygenation of the blood in the lungs and efficient removal of carbon dioxide. Oxygen is needed to break down the fats and lipids in the body in the process of energy conversion.

Perspiration during exercise gets rid of acids and toxic wastes near the skin surface and keeps the pores open for elimination. **The skin is an elimination organ, a "third kidney" so to speak, which helps keep the body free of toxic accumulations.** Toxins in tissues lower the metabolic rate and slow down the process of getting rid of fat.

Finally, some experts say that exercise depresses the appetite center, actually helping to control the urge to overeat. Possibly this is due to the more efficient digestion and assimilation that exercise stimulates, resulting in a lowered need and desire for food.

BEST FORMS OF EXERCISE

Walking briskly is the best all-around exercise, while swimming is the best exercise for those with back trouble. There are, however, many forms of exercise which are not suitable for overweight people, especially those 50 pounds or more over their ideal weight. We will present some special exercises for people with this condition.

Exercise should be regular, building up to at least one-half hour a day, preferably at the same time each day, strenuous enough to bring the pulse rate up, accelerate and deepen the breathing and bring on a light perspiration. For those 40 pounds or more overweight or those in poor physical condition, I recommend starting with no more than 10 minutes per day for the first two weeks, using easy stretching and bending exercises to get the body limber and to flex the joints. Don't strain and don't attempt to reach the perspiration point at first. Walking can be substituted. Walk four blocks or so each day the first three days and add two more blocks every three days until you are walking for a total of one-half hour. Then gradually increase the briskness of your walk until you are walking the same distance faster each day. Swimming can be substituted in a similar program. Start slow and easy, then build up in speed and distance gradually.

Horseback riding is very good for those who are in a position to do it once a week for an hour or so. Every muscle is the body is stimulated by the movement of the horse. The bowel and internal organs are flexed and toned, and the entire body is well oxygenated, which helps burn off fat calories. Keep in mind that horseback riding, or any other once-a-week form of exercise, should only be used along with a daily exercise program.

We do not get enough good from exercising once a week.

Fitness programs at health clubs are fine for some people but not for others. They can be very time consuming, considering the two-way drive and showering afterward, but if you are one of those who benefits from exercising with a group and are highly motivated by it, check it out with your doctor. I think many of the spa programs are beneficial, especially under supervision.

Be sure the kind of exercise you choose, the amount of time involved and the equipment, if any, will fit into your daily routine well enough to keep you motivated. The more you enjoy your exercise, the more likely you are to keep it up. Remember, music helps make exercise fun.

By equipment, I am referring to the various things you can buy at sporting goods stores, department stores and through some health food stores. These include indoor bicycle exercisers, bouncers that look like mini-trampolines, treadmills and gadgets with elastic bands to pull against. These can be very good, but make sure the equipment you choose is right for you before you buy.

My morning starts with skin brushing, exercising on my bouncer (mini-trampoline), to the music of three different tunes, then I take a brisk 15-minute walk in the hills near my Ranch. This fits me well, but you must find out what is best for you by trying out different exercises.

We should always start with warmup exercises, like simple stretches and bends, before getting into the active exercises. There are all kinds and degrees of aerobics. Some are quite strenuous. So, I want you to take it easy at first. Increase your efforts over a period of time; be good to your body.

A MUSICAL NOTE

Women, especially, love to exercise to music. Men do too, but I believe women are drawn more to dance by their natures. Women may be more deeply moved by music. So, I urge those who select exercises from the ideas in this chapter to do them to music, for greater benefits and higher motivation.

Music adds another dimension to exercise. No one can sit still when a lively polka is played. The feet tap, the legs move, the fingers tap, and the whole body gets into the rhythm and the spirit of the polka. One of the finest songs to use with beginner-level exercise is Lawrence Welk's MEMORIES. It is slow, but it moves nicely. The organ version of THE

HAPPY WANDERER is another. HOOKED ON CLASSICS or HOOKED ON SWING are wonderful to listen to while exercising.

Lawrence Welk deserves a great deal of credit for developing a musical style and beat that has moved many people off of their chair and onto the dance floor. I think he has drawn more people into dancing than any other orchestra leader, and dancing is wonderful exercise.

We find that the heavier person can do exercises to Lawrence Welk's music quite comfortably and enjoyably on a bouncer or rebounder (as the mini-trampoline is sometimes called) and I will describe some rebounder exercises you can do to music right after the section on *Stretching, Twisting and Bending Exercises.* If you start out slowly, carefully, it is not necessary to do any warmup exercises before getting on the bouncer because you will be warming up on it before getting into the more active side of exercising.

After your *skin brushing,* described below, I recommend that you start with Figure 8 exercises and a little stretching and bending for 5 minutes twice each day—before breakfast and before the evening meal. Gradually work up to a half hour of these exercises before changing to others. Don't let yourself get completely out of breath. Exercise only until you are feeling warm and perspiring lightly.

SKIN BRUSHING

I call the skin "the third kidney" because of its importance in eliminating acid wastes from the body. The skin is a living organ with blood and lymph vessels, nerves, oil glands and small muscles surrounding each hair and pore. Because dead skin cells build up on the skin, and because the muscles under the skin need stimulation, I recommend skin brushing as a method of stimulating, toning and cleansing that is not adequately done in taking a bath or shower. *SKIN BRUSHING AIDS REDUCING BY INCREASING THE RATE OF ELIMINATION.*

SKIN BRUSHING EXERCISE. Using a long-handled, vegetable bristle brush (not nylon bristles), scrub the body from neck to feet twice a day for about five minutes each time, as vigorously as is comfortable for you. Those who have very sensitive skin will have to go a little lighter on the brushing than others. Women should avoid brushing the breasts, and both sexes should use a softer brush on the face where the skin is more sensitive. We need to keep the skin active and stimulated. Brushing is done in any direction with a dry brush. We make new skin cells every 24 hours and *SKIN BRUSHING IS ESSENTIAL FOR HEALTHY SKIN AND ACTIVE ELIMINATION.*

FIGURE 8 EXERCISE SYSTEM FOR THE JOINTS

Fitness experts have a saying that goes *"Use it or lose it,"* and nowhere does this apply better than to the flexibility of the joints. We have to use them to keep them limber. There is another saying. *"You are as young as your joints,"* and this is something to think about. What can a person do once the joints become stiff?

We must have limber joints. If your joints are stiff now, you may have calcium deposits, so be careful. The diet I present at the end of the book, and my Health and Harmony Food Regimen which is to be used after you have reached your weight loss goal, will gradually bring any calcium deposits or spurs back into solution in the bloodstream. Meanwhile, go easy on the exercises, because moving the joints too much when there are calcium deposits may irritate the joints.

All Figure 8 exercises follow a circle pattern. The reason calcium spurs develop sometimes is because we don't use circular motion enough. When we walk or jog, our joints move back and forth, not around and around as they should. Figure 8s are *corrective exercises* and should be done every day.

You should understand by now that our weight-loss program in this book is designed to improve your health as you exercise and follow your diet. The two—diet and exercise—work together in *natural harmony.* Exercise without a proper diet is not wise.

OUR REDUCING PLAN IS DESIGNED TO WORK IN HARMONY WITH NATURE, AND THIS IS NOT WHAT MOST DIET PLANS DO. The Figure 8 Exercise System is the best system I know for the joints. They are carefully thought out and put together so you can get the greatest amount of good from them. We can also bring these exercises onto the bouncer if we want to. Figure 8 exercises are the best way I know to keep the joints limber and flexible. These exercises move the blood and lymph in the joint areas. They have been used by dancers for many years, and they will work just as well for you. Most people find them fun to do, especially to music. Repeat each exercise 3 to 6 times.

FIGURE 8 EXERCISE FOR THE KNEE JOINTS

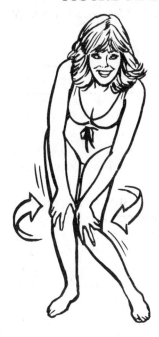

Move the knee joints in a circular motion by bending knees slightly, moving in circles or "figure 8" motion in each direction. Work up to 10 times each day (placing the hands on knees for balance is helpful). This knee exercise uses all sides of the joints not normally used, and keeps them pliable, limber and supple.

HIP JOINTS, FIGURE 8 EXERCISE

Stand with feet 6 to 8 inches apart and visualize a figure 8 on the floor. Stand in the center of the "8" and move hips and buttocks in circular or figure 8 motion in each direction. Work up to 6 to 8 times each direction. Make the figure 8 motion as large as possible to left and right sides. It is almost like the hula dance movement.

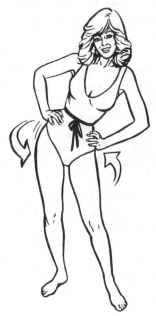

SHOULDER JOINTS, FIGURE 8 EXERCISE

Visualize a figure 8 around your shoulders. Move shoulders in figure 8 motion each direction. Lead with right and then left shoulders. Work up to 10 times each direction.

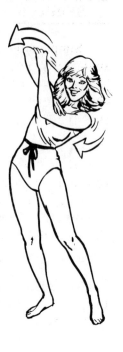

SPECIAL 8

A good figure 8 exercise follows one used by Fred Astaire, the well-known dancer and actor. He moves from side to side, lifting one shoulder and rising on his toes, then he follows the shoulder around in a circle. As he drops the other shoulder, he raises the arms and makes another figure 8. This exercise stretches the spine, coming up to compress the organs on the other side. Repeat 3 to 6 times on each side.

NECK, FIGURE 8 EXERCISES

This exercise is similar to the ancient Persian dance "neck loops." Look straight ahead. Do not look to either side. Slide the head straight over to the right side in the figure 8 or circular motion. The neck is over the shoulders, so to speak, a different movement than used in everyday movements and in different directions. Keep eyes and head looking straight ahead.

STRETCHING, TWISTING AND BENDING EXERCISES

Simple stretching, twisting and bending exercises can be done by anyone who does not have back problems. I will describe a few here to help you get started. Move slowly and gracefully, staying within the **comfort zone** with respect to how far you twist or bend and how much you stretch.

FLOOR TOUCHING

Raise both arms over your head and, bending at the waist, reach your hands toward your toes. If you are very heavy, this bend may seem more like a partial bow to a king, but don't push it. Only go as far as you can, 10 times. The eventual object is to be able to touch your toes on the floor without bending the knees.

AIRPLANE TWIST

Hold both arms straight out to the side like airplane wings. Keeping them straight, rotate right and left from the waist, twisting only as far as is comfortable. Do this 10 times.

SKY-REACH

Hold both arms straight up again. Pretend as if you were trying to grasp something above your head, just out of reach. You don't need to look up, just reach as high as you can, coming up on your tiptoes to reach a little higher. Breathe in with each stretch upward, exhale with each relaxation, coming down from tiptoe position but with the arms still extended up. Do 10 times.

STRETCH-REACH

Alternate arm stretches are a variant of number 3, using somewhat different muscles. In this exercise, raise both arms over the head again, but keep both feet flat on the floor. On an inward breath, stretch only the right arm upward, holding the spine as straight as possible, then exhaling as you bring the right arm back. Do the same with the left arm and continue alternating, 10 times each side.

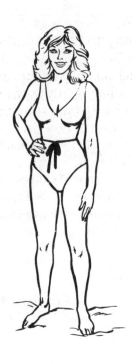
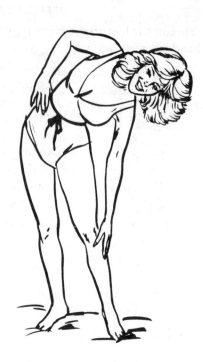

DOWN-STRETCH

Another side-stretching exercise starts by placing the right hand on the right hip, elbow out to the side, with the left arm straight down the left side, fingers extended. Carefully and gently extend the left hand down as far on the left leg as you can comfortably go. Don't try to over-reach. Do 10 times on the left, then 10 times on the right.

HIP ROTATION

Put both hands on hips. Holding the upper body straight and the legs straight together, rotate at the waist in a circular motion 5 times around to the left, 5 times around to the right in a circular motion.

DIVE-STRETCH

Spread the feet about 2 feet apart and bring the hands together above the head with as little elbow bend as possible, like a diver about to

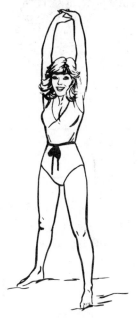

go off the diving board on a straight dive. Bending and rotating slightly at the waist at the same time, point the hands (together) first at the right foot, then between the two feet, then at the left foot, then swing back to the starting position to the count of 1-2-3-4. Don't try to bend or stretch to the point of discomfort. Eventually, you will be able to touch your toes and the floor but possibly not at first. Repeat 10 times.

(Alternative) Stand with knees slightly bent, feet 3 ft. apart. Raise your arms overhead, place hands together as if to dive into a pool. Bend slowly over from the hips, allowing knees to bend too, and reach as far back through legs as possible. Swing back into upright position, arms overhead again. Start slowly, increase speed as you go along. (10 times)

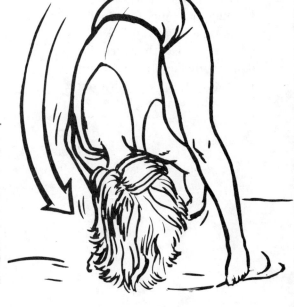

59

HALF SQUAT

Hands on hips, back erect, lower the buttocks about halfway to the knees, then come up again, breathing out on the down move, in on the up move. Do not attempt to go into a full squatting position. Halfway is sufficient. Repeat 10 times.

CHAIR EXERCISE SYSTEM
MORE STRETCHING AND BENDING

As in the case of the other exercises, these are more fun done to music. The only difference here is that you will be using a chair to help keep your balance while you do more stretching and bending.

SIDE-KICK

Place both hands on chair back, stand with feet together, keeping toes pointed, kick leg sideways (actually, this is more a quick leg "raise" than kick) bring it back and continue 10 times. Repeat with right leg. Raise the legs as high to the side as you can.

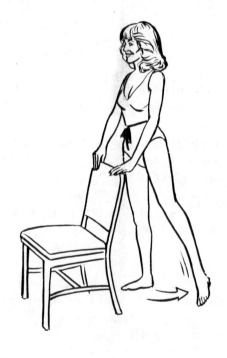

STRETCH AND SHIFT

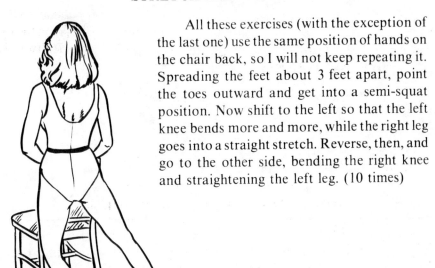

All these exercises (with the exception of the last one) use the same position of hands on the chair back, so I will not keep repeating it. Spreading the feet about 3 feet apart, point the toes outward and get into a semi-squat position. Now shift to the left so that the left knee bends more and more, while the right leg goes into a straight stretch. Reverse, then, and go to the other side, bending the right knee and straightening the left leg. (10 times)

CHAIR SQUATS

Same foot position as in the previous exercise, toes are pointed away from the body. Bending the knees as much as possible, lower the buttocks to the floor as far as you can, using the chair only to keep balanced. Then straighten up. Keep the spine straight and chin up. Do 10 repetitions—up, down, up, down and so on.

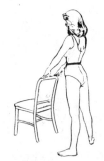

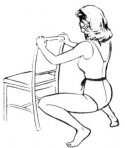

BACKWARD LEG LIFT

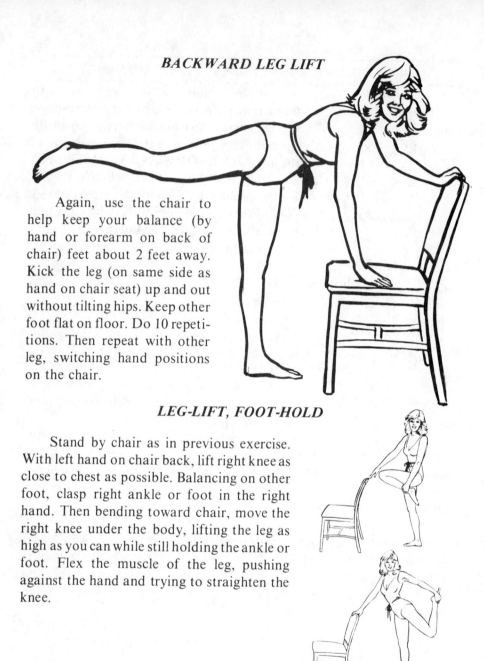

Again, use the chair to help keep your balance (by hand or forearm on back of chair) feet about 2 feet away. Kick the leg (on same side as hand on chair seat) up and out without tilting hips. Keep other foot flat on floor. Do 10 repetitions. Then repeat with other leg, switching hand positions on the chair.

LEG-LIFT, FOOT-HOLD

Stand by chair as in previous exercise. With left hand on chair back, lift right knee as close to chest as possible. Balancing on other foot, clasp right ankle or foot in the right hand. Then bending toward chair, move the right knee under the body, lifting the leg as high as you can while still holding the ankle or foot. Flex the muscle of the leg, pushing against the hand and trying to straighten the knee.

The benefit of all exercise is realized through rest. Always rest for at least 10 minutes after exercising, either lying down or sitting in a comfortable chair. A cup of Cleaver tea may be appropriate at this time.

REBOUNDER EXERCISE SYSTEM (TO MUSIC)

Rebounder exercises to music introduce a level and type of physical activity that most people can take. Three to five minutes on the rebounder is equal to a mile of jogging, and every muscle in the body is exercised *WITHOUT SUBJECTING THE JOINTS OR BONY STRUCTURES TO THE SUDDEN IMPACT SHOCK THAT TAKES PLACE WHEN RUNNING OR JUMPING ON A HARD SURFACE.*

Many years ago, after visiting an osteopath in Hawaii who had a full-sized trampoline in his backyard, I designed a minitrampoline for use by my patients long before the bouncers and rebounders so popular today were available.

We had a policeman at the Ranch who was on an early retirement due to an intervertebral disk problem that affected his back and neck, giving him a great deal of pain. I started him out on the bouncer with very easy exercises, gentle movements. He could do them without any problem, although he felt a little pain the day after his exercises. With my encouragement, he persisted and gradually increased the time and vigor of his exercises more and more. In a few weeks, his problem was corrected. This is what got me started on the rebounder exercises and showing my patients how to do them.

Rebounder exercises are actually tension-relaxation exercises. Our bodies tense as our feet land on the flexible cover of the rebounder and relax as we go into the air. This is what does our bodies so much good. The routine on the bouncer is a very important part of my own exercise regimen, and I enjoy this very much, always bouncing to music.

WE MUST BE KIND TO OUR JOINTS. The great thing about these rebounder exercises is that they are easy on the material that makes up the joints, and this is very important. Many exercises are harsh and jolting to the joints, compressing and stretching the soft inner material too much.

We must be kind to our joints because they say you are as young as your joints, and if they have been abused or if the diet is out of balance, they can become stiff, inflamed and painful.

The soft inner material of the joints is extremely sensitive to the acid/alkaline balance of the blood. If the blood is too acid, calcium spurs may develop. We must realize that incorrect diet and overexercise are harmful to the joint material.

Our exercises should never be so strenuous or overdone that more acids are produced than our diet and elimination channels can take care of, or the joints will be affected. We should never, in our lifetime, go beyond what our bodies can handle or we will find out there are consequences to our health. For this reason, diet and exercise should be well harmonized.

I usually start out with Lawrence Welk's *Memories,* then go to the organ version of *The Happy Wanderer,* and, last, something I like with a faster beat than the other two. You can substitute other music, but make sure the rhythm and tempo increase through the three songs or pieces you choose. It is best to record these three tunes on tape to run consecutively, so you can just turn on your tape recorder in the morning and get right into it. The time is about ten minutes for three pieces of music. You can increase the length of the music if you wish by adding other tunes later, after you are used to the ten minute starting program given here. I recommend the albums or tapes of *Hooked On Swing* or *Hooked On Classics.*

There are more than one set of exercises. Learn one—do it, then learn another and do this one. Then you can do 2, 3, 4, 5 combinations. Your daily exercise routine shouldn't take longer than 1/2 hour.

The main purpose of these exercises is to move the lymph and carry off the broken down products of fat metabolism. These movements firm the buttocks, help reduce the waist and strengthen the legs. Be inventive. Make up some of your own dance movements as you go along. The object is to use as many muscles as possible and to move as many of the joints as possible.

Turn on your music!

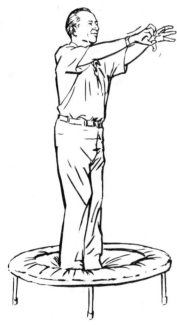

HANDS

Moving the feet in time with the music, let your body sway while flexing your fingers and hands with arms above head, down at your sides, extended like airplane wings, out in front of your body, behind your back. Work those fingers in time with the music in quick, flexing movements to exercise all the little muscles. You can continue the hand exercises in some of the other bouncer exercises, if you choose.

TOES AND ANKLES

Lift up on your toes, swing your heels in and out (toward one another, away from one another). Then bring the heels down and swing the knees (held closely parallel) in circles to the left and to the right.

KNEES

As you do these exercises, bend and straighten the knees, flex those knees, not removing your feet from the bouncer but "jogging" gently from the knees only.

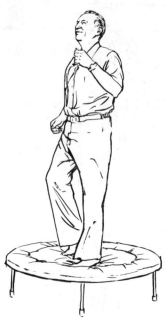

Try to follow as many figure 8 exercises as you can on the bouncer.

HULA HIPS

Move those hips in circular motion, then side to side, then front to back (thrusting the pelvis forward, then drawing it back), several times each motion. Move the arms in graceful hula-like motions, keeping the hands parallel, rolling the shoulders to work the upper body. Bring in the knee movements and the hand flexes.

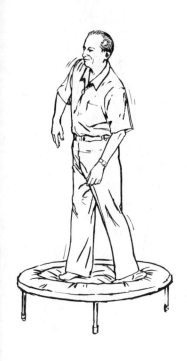

SHOULDER ROLLS

Drop hands to sides and rotate the shoulders alternately, left shoulder, then right shoulder, repeat, etc.; rotate in forward circles several times, then reverse circles, then do both shoulders at the same time, forward and reverse. Keep the legs going, the knees flexing, the hips swaying as you do this.

SWIMMING

Make swimming motions with the arms while keeping the feet, knees and hips moving—move the body continuously.

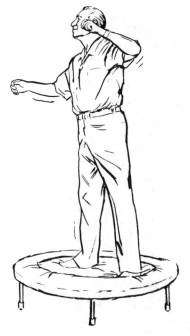

TWIST AND BEND

Twist the body from side to side several times, bend the body slightly forward, slightly backward several times.

NECK ROLLS

Move the neck from side to side, front to back, like a Persian dancer. Rotate hips in circles, the knees, the arms.

EYES (Not shown)

Hold the head still and make wide circles in the air in front of you, first with one hand, then the other, following your hands with the eyes. Repeat, closing the fist and making circles with one finger, following the finger with the eyes as you trace large circles clockwise then counterclockwise, first with one hand, then the other. Repeat 6 times each way. Then turn on the bouncer until you are squarely facing one wall. Again, holding the neck and head still, look from the upper right corner of the wall you are facing to the lower left corner, MOVING THE EYES ONLY. Shift the eyes to the upper left corner, then to the lower right. Repeat 6 times. Then shift the eyes to the right and do the same thing.

FIGURE 8 EXERCISES

The bouncer is a fine place to do the figure 8 exercises, and you may want to use them as part of your bouncer routine instead of doing them separately.

As the music shifts to the second tune, repeat the preceding exercises to the faster beat without lifting your feet from the bouncer. Do shoulder and arm movements like Fred Astaire or Ginger Rogers when they danced, especially the figure 8s with the arms and shoulders.

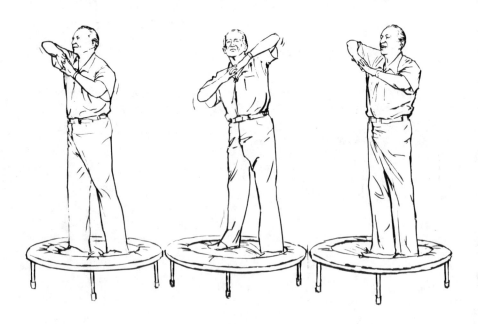

Do the hula hands, hula arms again. Move those feet! Repeat all hand and arm movements in the first four exercises. Move the hands in large circles in front of your face, one hand at a time, keeping your eyes on your hands without moving the neck. Do clockwise and counterclockwise circles. Keep moving in time to the music.

By the time the third and fastest piece of music comes on, you'll be warmed up enough to increase your activity level. When you increase the amount of time you spend on the rebounder, use it on this faster beat since you don't need any more of the warmups. Later, when you are able to use your rebounder to its limit, the more active exercise will increase your basal metabolism and continue to burn up more calories all day.

Repeat the movements as described in the first part of this section, but *vary the foot movements.*

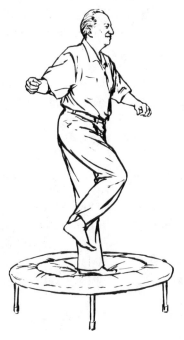

KNEE CROSSOVER
Cross the right knee over the left and bring it back. Repeat, crossing the left knee over the right 6 times each, alternating.

PIGEON-PENGUIN (Not shown)
Point toes together, heels apart, bounce. Then bring heels together, toes apart, bounce. Keep it up 6 times, alternating.

CHARLESTON (Not shown)
Do the Charleston, with small steps, so you can keep balanced; do 6 times.

69

KICKS →

Kick forward, one foot, then the other. When you kick, reach down toward the toes of the kicking foot with one hand, 6 times.

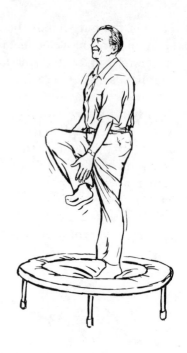

BELLYUP-BELLY DOWN
(Not shown)

As you bounce up, bring both hands to the lower-left abdomen and lift it a little as you go up and down, about 6 times. Then move the hands to the lower-right abdomen and repeat. Again, holding up the middle of the abdomen. You can do this with high jumps if you are comfortable in the process.

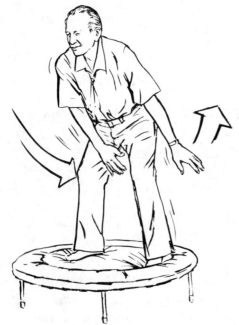

← ARM CIRCLES

Bend at waist, hands together, swing arms from side to side while bouncing on the mini-trampoline.

JUMP KICKS (GOOSE STEP)

This exercise helps to develop your balance. Kick your legs forward as if running. This is a bouncing exercise kicking legs forward.

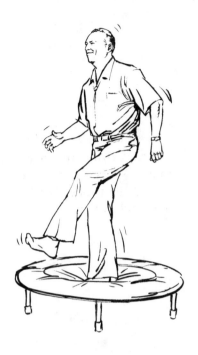

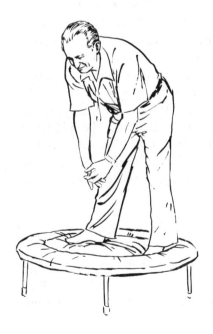

THE ELEPHANT

Clasp the hands, bend slightly forward and, with the feet apart, swing both arms to the left, then to the right, just as an elephant swings its trunk from side to side. The movement should be a graceful but energeteic arms-and-sholders stretch to one side then the other.

71

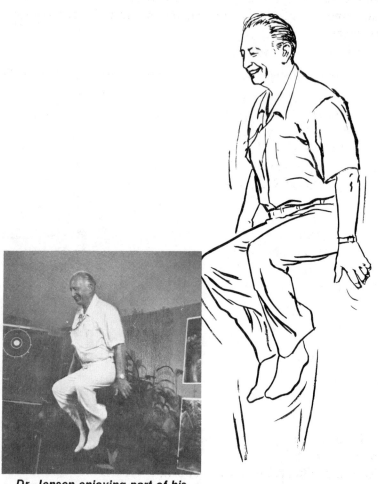

**Dr. Jensen enjoying part of his
daily bouncer routine.**

After you get used to these, dream up your own bouncer routine with any movements you like, including dance movements. When you are by yourself, be creative, let fantasies go into action. Just be aware of the flexibility and limited foot space of the bouncer. I can't begin to tell you all the nice things you can do on a bouncer, but I want to encourage you to make up some of your own exercises and have a good time with your bouncer!

Exercise is the most important process in taking care of lymphatic congestion, which is common in overweight people. The lymphatic system consists of the spleen, thymus, appendix, tonsils, lymph vessels, nodes and fluid. **The fluid moves by muscle contraction during movement.**

LYMPHATIC SYSTEM

FOODS. Green, leafy vegetables, watercress, celery, okra, apples.

DRINKS. Potato peeling broth, celery juice, blue violet tea, parsley juice, carrot juice, apple juice.

VITAMINS. A, C, choline, B-Complex, B-1, B-2, B-6, biotin, pantothentic acid, folic acid.

MINERALS. Potassium, chlorilne, sodium.

HERBS. Blue violet tea (leaves), chaparral, burdock, echinacea, blue flag, poke root, golden seal, cayenne, mullein, black walnut. (Best taken in extract form.)

If you are thirsty after exercising, add a crushed watercress tablet to your water or take an organic potassium tablet, so your body will not hold liquid. **This is especially important for those lymphatic types who retain water so easily.** Also, you may wish to take vitamin B-6 which has been recommended by health researchers to help keep the water down in the body. **Do not take more than 500 mg per day without talking to your doctor about it.**

There are plastic suits you can buy to increase perspiration while you exercise and afterward. Ask your doctor about this, since for some this may not be a safe procedure. **Perspiration is good for elimination of subcutaneous toxic material, but too much liquid loss can upset the chemical balance of the body.**

73

FLOOR EXERCISE SYSTEM

There are many good toning exercises that can be done lying down, but they are only for people who are able to get down and up from the floor without strain. If you are too heavy to safely do exercises on the floor, wait until you have shed enough pounds to do these more conveniently. Use other exercises until you are able to get down on the floor and back up without difficulty.

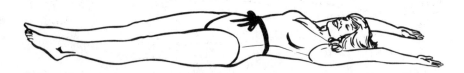

1. **Simple abdomen stretch.** Lying on your back, start with arms at the sides and lift them fully over the head, slowly, until they are flat on the floor above the head. Leave them there until a count of 10, then bring them back to the sides and start over. Do 10.

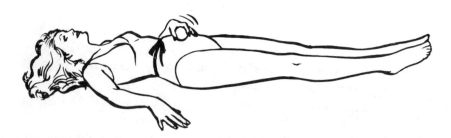

2. **Rubber ball exercise.** Lying on your back, head down on a slant board, or on the floor, roll a ball about the size of a tennis ball around on your abdomen with the palm of your hand. Use enough force so you can really feel it. This tones the bowel. Note any sore spots, and spend more rolling the ball over them. Like all slant board exercises, this one is particularly good for prolapsus of the transverse colon.

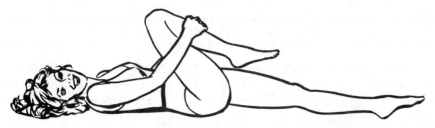

3. **Knee flex.** Lying on your back, draw the left knee as close to your chest as possible while breathing in, then return it to the floor while breathing out. Repeat with right leg. Do 10, each leg.

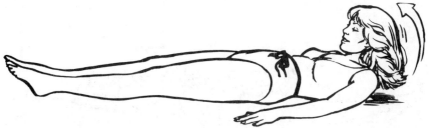

4. **Neck lift.** Lying on your back, try lifting your head slightly from the floor, tipping the chin toward your chest. Do not strain to do this. If you can't get your head off the floor at first, simply tense the muscles as if trying to do it, then relax. After a week, you should be able to get the head off the floor at least a little. Keep practicing. Start with 5 for the first week, work up to 10 by the end of the second week.

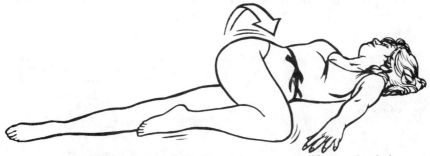

5. **Knee crossover, hip roll.** Do this one only if you don't have to strain. Lying on your back, bend the right knee and bring it over the left leg, rolling over partly on the left hip, while keeping the back on the floor and arms at sides, palms down to hold position. Only go as far as you can without straining, and do not roll over onto left side. Bring the right leg back to the floor, repeat with left leg and right hip. Do 5 each leg for the first week, then work your way up to 10 the second week.

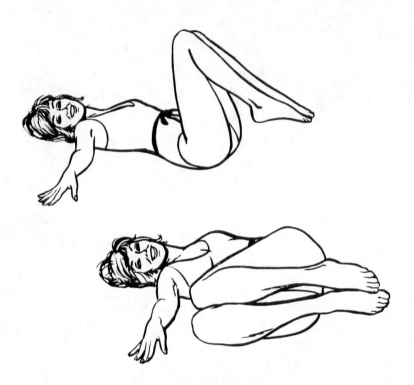

6. **Full hip rolls.** Lying on your back, put your arms out airplane style, palms to the floor for stability. Bring knees up as high as possible; then keeping knees bent and together, roll them to the left as far as you can without straining. Bring them back. Repeat on the right side. Start with 5 the first week and work up to 10 the second.

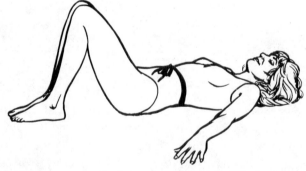

7. **Abdominal squeeze.** Lying on your back, lift the knees with feet flat on the floor. Knees should be touching. Take a breath, squeeze the knees together to the count of 1-2-3, then relax. Repeat for a total of 10.

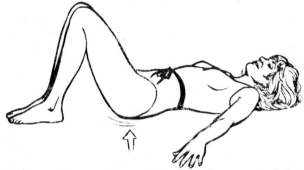

8. **Pelvic lifts.** With knees up and feet on floor, as in 6 & 7, press the lower back onto the floor while trying to lift and tighten the buttocks. Don't strain and don't try to lift your back up. If you don't get off the floor at first, don't worry. It will come. Squeeze the buttocks together as you lift. Start with 5, work up to 10 by the end of the second week.

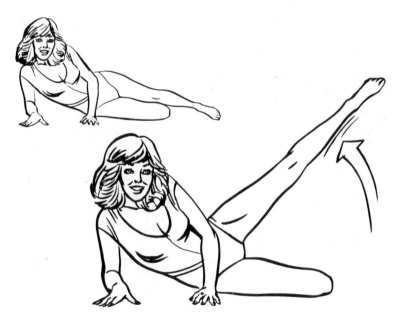

9. **Side leg lifts.** Roll onto your right side, get up on your right elbow and forearm and bend the right leg into an "L" at the knee for stability. Leave the top (left) leg straight, point the toes and try to lift the leg level with your hip or as high as is comfortable. Hold for a count of 1-2-3, let down and relax. Do this with both legs 5 times. Each week add another count, until you can hold each leg up to a count of 7.

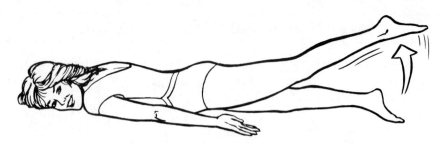

10. **More leg lifts.** Face and stomach down on the floor, lift one leg about 4-6 inches off the floor, hold briefly, then bring it down and repeat with the other leg. Inhale on the lift, exhale as you bring the leg down. Do four the first day, then add one more each day for each leg. If you can't get the legs off the floor at first, simply lift until you feel strain, then relax.

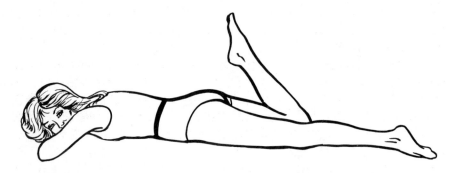

11. **Heel kicks.** Again lying face down on the floor, kick the heels back, one at a time, and try to touch the buttocks. Do five, each side.

SLANTING BOARD EXERCISE SYSTEM

Many times we don't realize that the body is underactive and overweight partly because the brain is not getting the proper blood circulation. This is extremely important because the brain is the symphony conductor that directs the activity of every organ, gland and tissue in the body, and if the brain is not fed right, the whole body suffers. The quickening force for every organ of the body comes from the brain, but people whose occupations cause them to sit or stand continually are sometimes unable to get the blood to the brain tissues because of inactive circulation and the counter force of gravity. Problems frequently formed are prolapsus of the transverse colon or prolapsed uterus (prolapsed means "dropped").

Slanting boards can be purchased at many sporting goods stores and department stores or they can be constructed by any "do-it-yourselfer." Basically, they consist of a padded board with a strap at one end to hold the ankles.

THE SLANTING BOARD IS THE BEST EXERCISE FOR GETTING BLOOD TO THE HEAD, FOR DRAWING A PROLAPSED COLON INTO PLACE, FOR RECTAL AND PROSTATE CONDITIONS, FOR UTERINE PRESSURE PROBLEMS, FOR IMPROVING CIRCULATION TO THE PELVIC ORGANS AND FOR RELEASING VENOUS BLOOD FROM THE LEGS. IT IS VERY GOOD FOR DEVELOPING TONE IN THE TISSUES OF AN ENLARGED ABDOMEN.

CAUTION

DO NOT attempt to use the slant board until or unless you are able to get up and down easily from the floor. Those with heart conditions, high blood pressure, internal bleeding or other serious health conditions should consult their doctors about using the slanting board. Wait at least 2 hours after eating to use the board.

SUGGESTED SLANT BOARD EXERCISES

Follow instructions carefully. You can feel relaxed, refreshed and invigorated quickly by stimulating circulation to all parts of the body. Do not try to do too much at first. Take on more exercises gradually. Do not attempt exercises that might endanger physical condition. If in doubt, have a physical checkup.

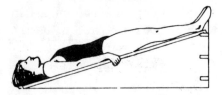 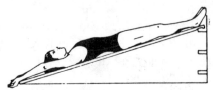

1. Lie full length, allowing gravity to helpl the abdominal organs into their position. Lie on board at least 10 minutes.

2. While lyng flat on back, stretch the abdomen by putting arms above head. Bring arms above head 10-15 times. This stretches the abdominal muscles and pulls the abdomen down toward the shoulders.

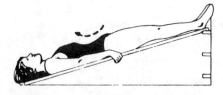 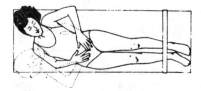

4. Pat abdomen vigorously with open hands. Lean to one side then to the other, pattig the stretched side. Pat 10-15 times on each side. Bring the body to a sitting position, using the abdominal muscles. Return to lying position. Do this 3-4 times, if possible. Do only if doctor orders.

3. Bring abdominal organs toward shoulders while holding breath. Move the organs back and forth by drawing them upward, contracting abdominal muscles, then allowing them to go back to a relaxed position. Do this 10-15 times.

SUGGESTED SLANT BOARD EXERCISES (Continued)

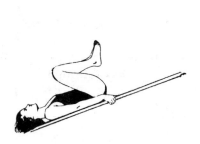

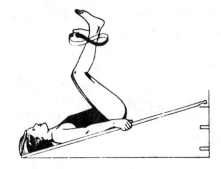

5. Bend knees and legs at hips. While in this position: (a) turn head from side to side 5 or 6 times; (b) lift head slightly and rotate in circles 3 or 4 times.

6. Lift legs to vertical position, rotate outward in circles 8 or 10 times. Increase to 25 times after a week or two of exercising.

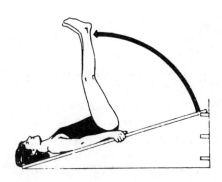

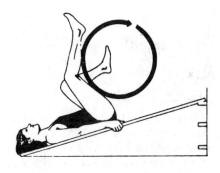

7. Bring legs straight up to a vertical position and lower them to the board slowly. Repeat 3 or 4 times.

8. Bicycle legs in air 15 to 25 times.

THREE SHAPING AND FIRMING EXERCISES FOR WOMEN

We find that some people profit more by variety of exercises while others do better with only a few simple ones. The following exercises, if faithfully used, will do more to firm up and tone the body than most exercise programs. *REDUCING THE CALORIE INTAKE OF FOODS LOWERS THE WEIGHT, WHILE CORRECT EXERCISE RESTORES THE RIGHT FIRMNESS AND PROPORTION TO THE BODY.*

These exercises should be done first thing in the morning, after drinking a glass of water with a teaspoon of liquid chlorophyll. Wear pajamas, sweat suit or an exercise outfit of some kind. *It is best to keep them up for three months at least.*

ARM AND LEG SHAPE-UP EXERCISE

For firming the arms from shoulders to wrists, and the upper legs, calves and ankles.

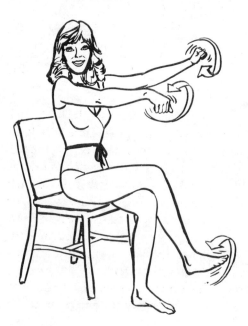

Sit in a straight-backed chair, preferably without arms. Cross the right leg over the left at the knee; bring up right foot until knee is almost straight. Extend both arms out straight in front of you and make tight fists. As you rotate your right foot from the ankle in circles to the right, rotate the right fist in a circle to the right and the left fist in a circle to the left. Keep the weight of the right leg resting on the left knee, but keep that foot up. The foot rotations may seem awkward but keep them up. *You'll get better at it.*

(Continues next page.)

82

After 10 repetitions, reverse the direction of rotation of the right foot and the two arms and do 10 more. Then, place the left leg over the right knee and repeat the whole process. Increase rotations by 5 each month (in each direction with each foot).

BODY FIRM-UP EXERCISE

For firming the stomach, strengthening the abdominal muscles, firming the neck, shoulders and arms, straightening the spine, eliminating swayback and lifting the breasts.

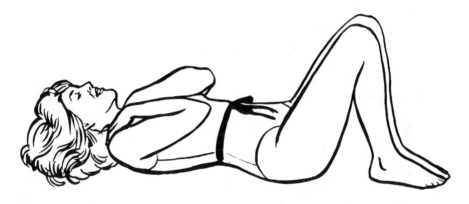

Lie on your back on the floor. (For all floor exercises, lie on a thick rug or use an exercise mat.) Raise the knees and bring the feet back toward the buttocks as far as you can without discomfort, keeping the feet flat on the floor. With elbows hugging your sides, touch each hand to the shoulder on its side, right hand to right shoulder, left hand to left shoulder. Now sweep the hands in a circular motion, out and up along the floor, until the two hands come together above the head. At the same time you raise the arms, straighten out the legs. When you've reached the endpoint, stretch the hands up a little higher, the feet down a little farther, so you feel the muscles stretching throughout the body.

Return arms and legs to original position, then repeat 10 times each day for the first week. Add 2 repetitions per week until you're up to 30.

CHANGING THE BOTTOM LINE EXERCISE

This is an interesting exercise, designed to take inches off the derriere and make lovely curves to replace the bulges. Now, this is not so much an exercise as a principle of exercise for this part of the body, and there are several different ways we can do it.

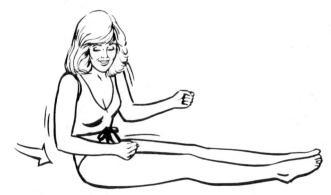

The first variation is called *the walk*. Sit on the floor, legs outstretched in front of you, feet together, arms at sides, elbows bent as if you were about to start a race. Twist the body somewhat sharply to the left, then to the right, *walking* the buttocks forward as you twist the torso and arms right—left—right—left, and so on. Keep it up for 2 minutes the first week, and extend to 5 minutes (or more) in 3 months.

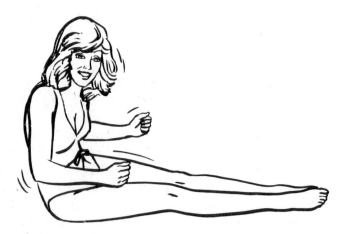

The second variation, modeled on the first, involves the same movements, only remaining in place and simply *rocking* from side to side, not *walking* forward.

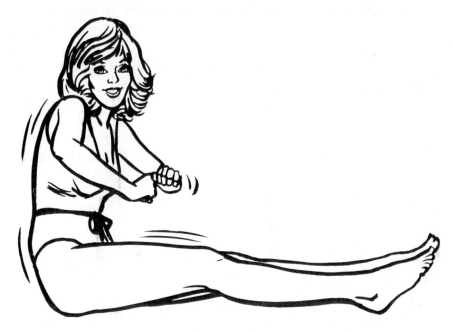

The third variation, another **rocker,** calls for sitting on the floor in the same position, extending the arms out sideways like airplane wings, then wagging one **wing** at a time as you rock from one side to the other.

Since the second and third variations are easier, try to keep them up for five minutes if you opt to do them instead of the first, and increase the time you take doing them each week.

This is basically a three month regimen, but it may take less for some and more for others to firm up the body.

SYSTEM FOR IMPROVING THE REAR VIEW (AND THIGHS)

The thighs and rear are the most difficult for many women to keep slender and toned as they would like. But, here are some exercises especially designed for a two-month program to get the flab off the buttocks and upper thighs.

Some physical fitness experts say that spot reducing is impossible because any exercise uses up calories which are more or less uniformly taken from all over the body, but I have seen too many examples of successful spot reducing to believe that. I feel that the caloric demand takes place in the tissue being exercised, and that localized fatty deposits are removed first.

Many times we find that an enlarged "rear view" is associated with lower back problems, so we have to take care of this part of the anatomy as we do the rest of the body. We find out that a tendency to gain weight in the lower half of the body but not the upper half (or vice versa) can be due to a pituitary imbalance, and some patients report that the Chinese herb Dong quai has helped women with this problem, while ginseng has helped men. The herbs must be used along with exercise for best results, to help balance the body proportions.

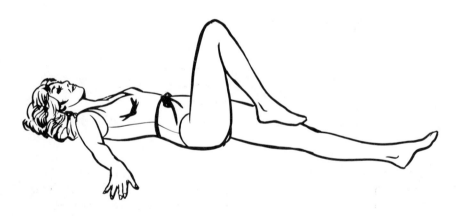

1. **Hip roll.** Lie flat on your back, arms at side, palms on the floor, legs out straight, then draw the left knee up toward your chest. Keeping the upper torso flat against the floor, leaving the right leg straight, twist

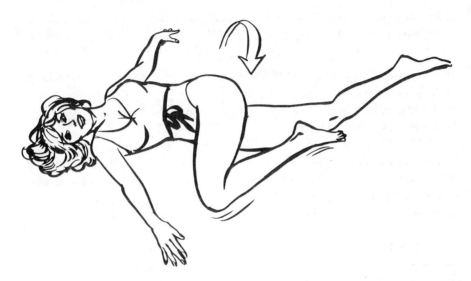

the hips to the right until the left knee touches the floor. Repeat 10 times and do the same thing with the right leg and knee.

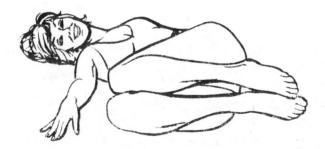

2. **Hip roll.** (Variation) When you can do the first exercise easily, try bringing both knees up and doing the same thing—roll hips and swing knees to the right, not touching the floor, then to the left, 10 repetitions to start with. The exercise is slightly easier if you turn your head in the opposite direction as you are swinging your knees. Work up to 25 of these in two months by adding 2 repetitions each week.

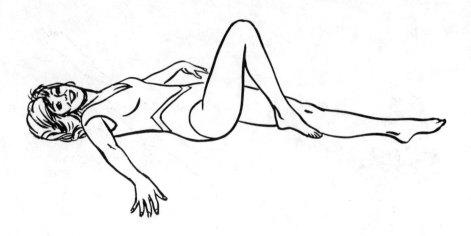

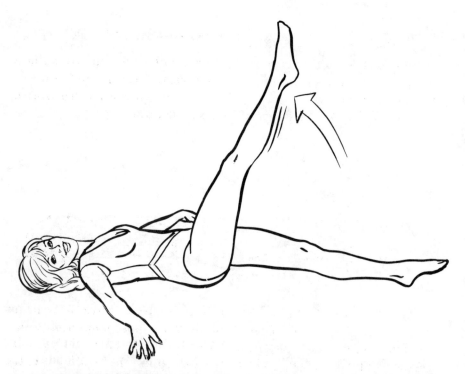

   3. **Straight kicks, lying down.** On the back, arms at sides, right knee up, left foot flat on the floor, smoothly kick the right leg straight up (as high as you can). Repeat 10 times. Then do the same with the left leg, 10 times. Work up to 30 in two months.

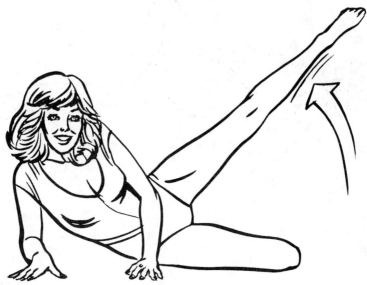

4. **Flipper-flaps.** Lie on one side and support your upper torso in an upright position, while bending the underneath knee into an "L-shape.". Now begin lifting the top leg—up, down, up, down. Start with 6, work up to 18 each side. Vary by keeping top leg bent during lifts.

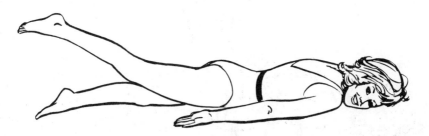

5. **Leg lifts, reverse.** Turn over on your stomach, arms at sides, palms face up on floor. Turn your head to your most comfortable side, separate your feet six inches. Take a deep breath. Lift the right leg, point the toe, contract the buttocks, count 1-2-3, let out the breath, lower the leg, relax the buttocks. Keep the pelvis flat on the floor throughout the exercise. Switch to left leg and do the same to the count of 1-2-3, exhaling as you lower the leg and relax the buttocks. Start with 6 on each leg, increase 3 each week to 30 repetitions.

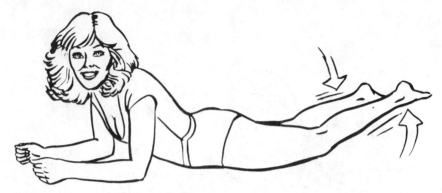

6. **Swim kick.** Lying on the stomach, support your upper torso partly on the forearms and look straight ahead, raising the feet about a foot off the floor. Tighten the buttocks and kick as though swimming, 20 repetitions each leg, working your way up to three minutes of rapid kicking in two months.

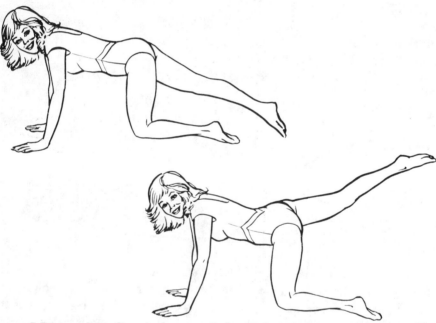

7. **Pony kick.** Get down on all fours, hands far enough apart for comfortable support, knees about a foot apart. Extend the left leg behind you, off the floor, knee slightly bent. Now lift and lower the leg, smoothly, but rapidly, 10 times. Then the other leg, 10 times. Build up to 30 in 2 months.

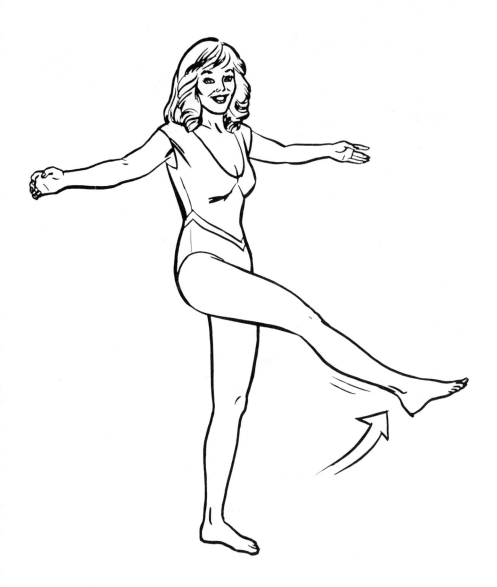

8. **Erect-Kick.** Standing up straight, feet together, kick as high forward as you can with the right leg, 10 times. Repeat with left leg. Don't jerk or use too much strength the first week. Add five kicks each week, and aim for kicking above your head.

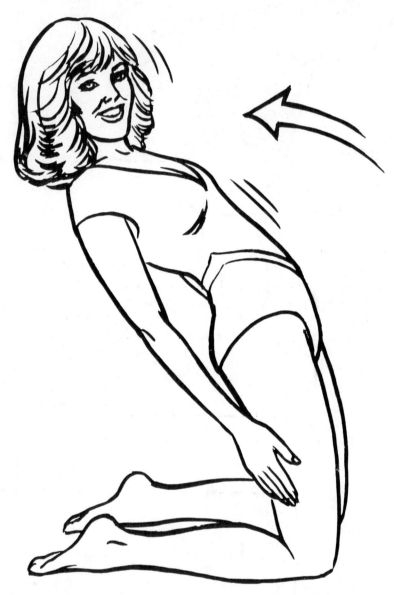

9. **Teetering.** This one is fun. Get on your knees, spine erect, palms on thighs. Holding the head and body straight, tense the buttocks, inhale deeply, and teeter back as far as you can hold without straining. Hold to a slow count of 1-2-3-4-5. Breathe out and go back to a relaxed upright position. Do 5 and try to build up to 20 in two months.

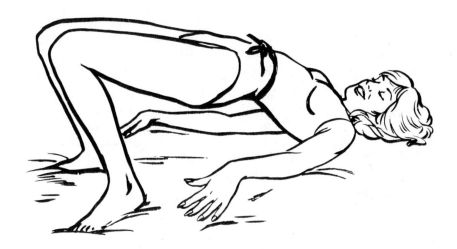

10. **Arch-lift.** On your back, on the floor, arms at sides, palms down, lift the knees and bring both feet back until they are flat on the floor. Take a deep breath as you raise the buttocks, arching your pelvis and lower back off the floor. Go only as far as you can without straining, and hold to the slow count of 1-2-3-4-5, before slowly coming back down. Do 4 of these the first week, working up to 10 in two months. Try to get a little farther off the floor after the second week, and as you improve, increase the count to 7, then 9, then 11, etc.

11. Finish with 10 minutes of bouncing on a mini-trampoline, calisthenics or dance movements to fast music with a good beat.

Different people progress at different rates. If you like these exercises, but are not quite sure where you want to be in two months, keep them up.

OTHER WAYS TO STAY FIT

There are many types of exercises and many ways to get exercise, such as gardening, weeding, washing windows, mowing the lawn, washing the car, taking the stairs instead of the elevator, riding a bicycle to a nearby market to get a few things instead of taking the car. *Think about it.* Most of us drive too much. *Legs were made to walk with, and we can all benefit from as much walking as possible.*

Our legs are the pumps that drive the venous blood back to the heart, and using them often is the key to good circulation and cardiovascular health. Blood tends to stagnate in the leg veins if we don't get enough exercise, and this may lead to varicose veins. Dr. Paul Dudley White, the late President Eisenhower's heart specialist, often pointed out that we die from our feet up. He once said that if you have flabby legs, you will have a flabby brain—a lighthearted comment, but one with more than a grain of truth in it. There is considerable evidence to indicate that firm, well-exercised legs lead to a long life, and this is what I saw in the Hunza Valley of Pakistan where men over 100 years old walked up and down mountain paths each day to work in the fields on the terraced hillsides.

Check out the nature trails closest to where you live and visit them with a friend or two. Make sure they are safe and use them as often as you can. If you live by a beach, lake or forest, walk where your eyes can feast on beauty. ***Beautiful sights are the vitamins and minerals of the mind.***

Fresh air and sunshine are vital elements of health, too, and one way to get more of them is to go bicycling or hiking in the country. Backpacking and jogging are wonderful forms of exercise, but strenuous unless you are in shape. Horseback riding exercises most of the muscles of the body. Camping is a light exercise form of recreation, but plan meals carefully in advance. It is all too easy to build up a great appetite and overeat.

The better the physical condition we are in, the more efficiently the body works, and the trimmer we stay—as long as we remain aware and in control of what goes in the mouth.

NURTURING OF THE SKIN AND CARE OF WRINKLES

Wrinkles in the skin have many causes—poor diet, lack of certain vitamins and minerals, dryness due to exposure to sun and wind, flabby muscle structure beneath the skin and habitual patterns of facial expression. For example, frowning is said to involve a pattern of facial muscle stretching that encourages a particularly unattractive wrinkle pattern over the years. Another cause of wrinkles is loss of subcutaneous fat due to weight reduction. These wrinkles tend to go away as new skin replaces the old, but we can do much to hasten the process.

We find that a healthy diet sometimes brings on elimination through the skin—unsightly blemishes and various types of eruptions as the body is being cleansed of old toxic wastes and catarrh. Worry and anxiety are also believed to contribute to skin troubles. Once the cleansing is over, the skin troubles will vanish and the skin will be softer and more beautiful than ever.

The skin is basically a silicon organ, and foods richest in silicon, such as alfalfa sprouts and rice polishings, will enhance its texture. The skin needs vitamin A especially but also B-complex, vitamins E and F.

Iodine foods are needed, and one of the foods highest in iodine is Nova Scotia dulse, a member of the seaweed family. The Japanese eat over 70 varieties of seaweed because it is rich in minerals, including trace minerals needed in very small amounts by the body. Chemical analysis of a sample of kelp showed the following mineral contents, all vital to health.

CHEMICAL CONTENTS OF KELP

Iodine	0.18%	Magnesium	0.74%
Calcium	1.05%	Sodium	3.98%
Phosphorus	0.34%	Chlorine	13.07%
Iron	0.37%	Manganese	0.0015%
Copper	0.0008%	Sulphur	1.0%
Potassium	11.15%		

Skin brushing with a natural bristle brush not only hastens skin elimination, removes dead skin cells and stimulates elasticity and tone in the underlying new skin structure, but it also helps get rid of cellulite, the layer of subcutaneous fat that tends to pucker the skin on overweight or physically inactive women.

Regular forms of exercise will tone the muscle tissue underlying the skin and improve blood circulation to the skin areas, but there are several exercises that are especially helpful in reducing or eliminating facial wrinkles.

FACIAL EXERCISE SYSTEM FOR SKIN TONING

It is best to do these exercises 10 times, 3 times each day, but it is also good to practice them in odd moments during the day. Either make sure no one is around or tell people what you're doing so they won't think you're strange.

WRINKLES UNDER THE EYES. First look straight ahead, then, keeping the head in that position, look up at the sky or ceiling and wink 5 times, rest, wink 5 times more, etc. This will help get rid of wrinkles in the lower eyelids. In the usual way of winking, only the upper eyelids get the exercise.

CROW'S FEET at the corners of the eyes can be helped by raising the lowering the eyebrows which also exercises forehead muscles. Also, rolling the fingertips over the wrinkled area behind the eyes (sides of forehead), twice a day will help. Any time you can bring cold water to the facial wrinkles, you will help tone the muscles underneath them.

TEMPLE AND FOREHEAD MUSCLES are also strengthened by squeezing the eyes tightly shut. An inverted cold spoon on the eye will many times help wrinkles disappear. Do this many times a day.

TO TONE THE CHEEKS AND MUSCLES around the mouth, there are several wonderful exercises. One is to pucker the lips, then stretch the corners of the mouth wide, as in grinning. Another is to pucker the lips, then move them alternately to the left and to the right. A third is to open the mouth wide, hold it open and move the lips. A fourth is to lift the cheek muscles, as in squinting the eyes, then relax them.

CHIN WRINKLES are helped by raising the lower lip above the upper lip and bringing it back to normal position.

TO HELP SMOOTH THROAT WRINKLES, tilt the head back as far as possible, then pucker the lips and wrinkle up your nose at the same time.

THE HONEY PAT is another special technique for getting rid of wrinkles and helping remove blackheads and whiteheads from the skin. Pour a little honey in a saucer, dip your fingers in it and apply it to the face, drawing the facial skin and muscles out with the sticky honey. This exercises the muscles and pores and helps develop the tone of the underlying tissue. Do this 10 times daily for two months, together with skin brushing exercises.

In general, I do not believe in using lotions, creams and salves, but I feel that apricot kernel oil is very soothing to the skin, and I feel it is the best.

Keep in mind that skin cells are replaced very rapidly and the smoothing of wrinkles from loss of fatty tissue will not take long, especially if aided by the preceding exercises.

A FINAL NOTE OF ADVICE ON EXERCISE

There are many kinds of exercise, and all have their special benefits. Pick the system that will help tone the part of your body that needs it the most, and stay with it until you feel you are ready to move on with another system.

7

My Health and Harmony Food Regimen

Sooner or later, we have to get away from diets and turn to a right way of eating, a right way of living. I don't even like the word "diet." It conjures up thoughts of hospitals and doctors and nutritionists with special meal plans tailored for people who are seriously ill. When we stop and think about it, a diet is sometimes a deliberately imbalanced eating regimen designed to counter an imbalanced health condition. But, it can also be imbalanced through ignorance or carelessness.

Here I am teaching a balanced way of living and we find out if we have a balanced way of living we don't have to cut back on the food we should have. A good food regimen isn't a matter of always eating the foods we like, since there are many foods that are good for us, and we can learn to like them. For instance, I didn't like avocados to begin with but I like them now. A lot of people don't like okra, but it is a wonderful food. So is asparagus. We should learn to appreciate and take greater pleasure in a much wider variety of foods.

For example, you have been on a weight-gaining diet or you probably wouldn't be reading this book. I was on a weight-gaining diet once—four milkshakes a day with whipped cream and a cherry on top— and I almost died from it. There are coffee and donut diets, meat and potato diets, hamburger and french fry diets, juice diets, cabbage and peanut diets—all kinds of diets—and they are killing the people who eat them. So, it makes a great deal of sense to get off diets, to get away from imbalanced food habits.

As I have said before, weight loss and weight management are like learning to play the piano. You have to practice, practice, practice to do it well. In the learning stages you will make mistakes but never mind—keep practicing. The skill you gain in practicing, with constant application, will become beautiful music. Practic makes perfect, as they say. The day will come when playing will not require such concentration and effort, because it will be natural to you. With perseverence the "new you" will emerge as surely as the sun rises in the morning.

WHAT YOU DON'T KNOW CAN HURT

Most Americans develop food preferences during childhood, from the patterns of food, cooking and preparation used in the parents' home. Teenage girls may learn a little more about cooking and nutrition in high school, but since it isn't a "real life" situation, such facts are often quickly forgotten. Newly married wives try to discover the sorts of things their husbands like to eat, then incorporate these into the menu plan of their new home life. When we stop and think about it, most food decisions made at the supermarket and in the kitchen are not centered around nutritional value, but around cost, taste, convenience, ease of cooking, advertising, heresay and tradition.

The first thing I want to tell you is that the average American eats far too much milk and wheat. A government survey showed that 54% of the American diet is made up of these two products—25% milk products and 29% wheat products. Both are fattening, especially in those quanities. I believe that the pasteurization of milk and the refining of wheat into flour alter both foods in such a way that they are more fattening, more difficult for the body to handle than in their natural, whole state. Wheat is one of the most fattening of the grains. People who have this much wheat and milk are wheat-logged and milk-logged. All allergy doctors tell you this is a high catarrh-producing diet, and allergies follow after this high amount of catarrh. We find that catarrh is associated with practically all allergy conditions, bronchitis, coughs, colds, flu, pneumonia, hay fever, asthma and so forth.

The two foods, milk and wheat, should not total more than 6% of all the foods taken. If we could get it down to 6%, we would balance our diet and stay away from many of our weight problems. Our **Health and Harmony Food Regimen** will take care of most of our health problems.

When the kitchen is ruled by ignorance, the dining room table leads to the doctor's office and to the doctor bills that naturally follow.

As we look at how we are living in the USA, especially over the last 30 years, we see that diet and trends in buying foods as related to the way foods are advertised may be the reason why over 40% of the people are obese. The three foods advertised most are wheat, milk and sugar. The amount of these three foods in the average diet violates the Law of Excess; for example, the American diet consists of 29% wheat, 25% milk and at least 9% sugar. If we add up these percentages, the total is 63%. I wonder if we are squeezing out the very foods that would keep us at a normal weight. These three foods are high-calorie foods and because they are overused, I am sure they are contributing to the overweight problem in America. These three foods are contributing most to the ill health in America including the overweight problem. We have had patients who cut out only these three foods and used substitutes instead, resulting in considerable loss of excess pounds. In early all cases where people have stopped using these three foods in excess, we have found very good results in overweight cases. I believe that 63% is too much, and these foods should run only about 6% in our total diet. This is especially necessary when we are trying to get well when we are going through an adjustment period.

The cure for ignorance is knowledge, and I think it is wonderful that nature is so generous and willing to point us in the right direction. My **Health and Harmony Food Regimen** is taken from nature's kitchen. You and your family can live well and be healthy on it.

CLEANING OUT THE CUPBOARDS AND PANTRY

If we want to clean out the body, we can go on an elimination diet. But if we want to keep it clean, we have to clean out the cupboards and pantry. We have to stop eating wrong foods before eating the right foods will do us much good.

The first things to get rid of are white flour and white sugar—the refined carbohydrates. These are hard on the pancreas, adrenals, liver, kidneys and bowel, and are probably even more responsible for obesity than fatty foods. We must have fiber in our foods from the complex carbohydrates, the fresh fruits and vegetables, whole grains, etc. Instead of sugar, use a little honey now and then for sweetening, or use naturally sweet fruits and dried fruits like figs, dates, raisins, apricots and so forth.

It is better to use herb seasonings than spices, and you will be surprised at the delightful flavors you can get with herbs. Use cayenne pepper instead of black pepper, which is hard on the liver. Cayenne pepper is good for the digestion and circulation.

Cut back on use of milk products, since many Americans are milk-logged, which can be catarrh producing, constipating and definitely fattening. Yogurt and kefir are better for those over 40 who have a harder time digesting milk products, best when they are raw. Clabbered milk is also easily digestible.

I feel it is to your advantage to eliminate all fatty meats and pork from the diet. Cut back on the use of beef and substitute more fish and poultry instead. Fish should have fins, scales and white meat. Salmon is also very good. Meat should be baked or broiled, never fried. Don't use meat fat (such as bacon grease or lard) for any cooking purpose.

AVOID coffee, tea and all soft drinks. Caffeine is hard on the nerves, sugar is a nutritional disaster and artificial sweetners are considered harmful by many scientists. For example, saccharine, a coal tar derivative, has been linked to cancer. Herb teas and natural coffee substitutes are much better for you. Since this regimen includes more fresh fruits and vegetables, you will be getting more water from them and you don't need to drink as much liquid with or between meals as on your former diet.

You may be using food items I have not listed here, but which are valueless or harmful. Read the label, think about the product, ask questions. You should evaluate what you intend to put into your body. Use whole grain flours for baking, but try to cut down on baked goods and on the use of wheat products in general. Most Americans eat far too much wheat, and a wheat-logged body can become imbalanced to the point of being susceptible to allergies and obesity.

Throw out the table salt and do not buy substitutes that taste like it unless they are natural. Salt has been linked to hypertension and water retention; it may be the chloride in it that is causing the trouble. There are vegetable seasonings, broth powders and herbs that make lovely flavor enhancers for vegetables and proteins. They are good for us, without harmful side effects, and some taste "salty."

Iceberg lettuce has so little food value that leaf lettuce is by far the better buy. Why waste the money? Most citrus is picked green for shipping, so I recommend against it. If you can get tree-ripened citrus, it is all right to eat it, sliced in sections, for the bulk value. There are many other fruits in season for you to eat and you should have a variety. Fresh sun-ripened fruits are best.

Throw out most packaged and canned products, and anything else that has been processed or contains chemical additives. Processing reduces food value and increases price, and, you are paying for labor—not increased worth. Most canned and packaged foods contain salt, sugar or both, in addition to chemical preservatives, colorings, flavor enhancers, texturizers, moisturizers and various other chemicals. These are unnatural to the body, and untold harm may result from them over the long term. Packaging, canning and chemicals add to the cost of the food as well. Additives react most strongly with the fat cells, where drugs and toxic materials are stored.

FOOD LAWS TO FOLLOW

Nature has given us bodies that respond best to foods in certain combinations and amounts, as listed below. A rule-of-thumb for eating is, never eat until you have a keen desire for simple food. Don't eat if you are ill, emotionally upset or chilled. Eat only small portions of easily digested foods if you are tired or fatigued.

The family should eat at the same table at the same time, keeping conversation pleasant. The table is no place for discipline, scolding, insults or verbal abuse of any kind. Food should be adequately chewed—especially raw vegetables and starches. One way to discourage eating too rapidly is to put the fork down between bites. Teach your children that it is always healthier to eat too little than too much.

FOOD LAWS

1. DAILY DIET

Daily diet should be 80% alkaline and 20% acid foods, as shown on the Acid/Alkaline Chart. This means you will select 8 alkaline foods and 2 acid foods daily.

2. NATURAL

Fifty percent (50%) and sixty percent (60%) of the food eaten should be raw. If, for any reason, you can't follow this law, take 1 teaspoon of wheat bran or psyllium husks after each meal. This will take care of the fiber needed in your diet.

3. PROPORTION

Six (6) vegetables, 2 fruits, 1 starch and 1 protein daily. (This keeps your daily food total 80% alkaline, 20% acid.) This matches what the blood should be.

4. VARIETY

Vary proteins, starches, vegetables and fruits from meal to meal and day to day. Know 7 good proteins, 7 good starches, 7 good salad dressings, 7 herb teas—so you get variety.

5. EXCESS

Excess in one or a few foods is to be avoided because thils creates imbalance in the body. Wheat, milk and sugar are the greatest offenders I know, and they all contribute to weight problems. **EXCESS** eating of all foods, even in a balanced eating regimen, leads to the development of fatty tissue, a condition of imbalance within the body. Any form of excess leads to imbalance of some kind.

6. DEFICIENCY

Deficiency in foods containing the chemical elements, vitamins and other nutrients causes imbalance in the body and, in general, prevents tissue repair and rebuilding. This is especially important with regard to inherently weak organs of the body, which are unable to hold nutrients and chemical elements as well as normal tissues. The most common deficiencies I have encountered are calcium, sodium, silicon and iodine, and these should be obtained from foods or supplements derived from foods.

7. COMBINATIONS

Separate proteins and starches: one at lunch, one at dinner. Have fruit for breakfast and, if desired, at 3 pm.

If reducing, have two protein meals and only one starch meal in the regular regimen.

ACID-ALKALINE CHART

The following table of foods is from Ragnar Berg of Germany.

Foods preceded by the letters "AL" are alkaline forming.   Foods preceded by the letters "AC" are acid forming.

Column No. 1
Nonstarch Foods

AL	Alfalfa
AL	Asparagus
AL	Beans (wax)
AL	Beet leaves
AL	Cabbage (white)
AL	Carrots
AL	Cauliflower
AL	Chickory
AL	Corn
AL	Dandelions
AL	Endive
AL	Horseradish
AL	Kohlrabi
AL	Lettuce
AL	Okra
AL	Onions
AL	Parsley
AL	Peas (fresh)
AL	Radishes
AL	Savory
AL	Sorrel
AL	Soybean (products)
AL	Summer squash
AL	Turnips
AL	Artichokes
AL	Beans (string)
AL	Beets (whole)
AL	Broccoli
AL	Cabbage (red)
AL	Carrot tops
AL	Celery knobs
AL	Cocunut
AL	Cucumbers
AL	Eggplant
AL	Garlic
AL	Kale
AL	Leek
AL	Mushrooms
AL	Olives (ripe)
AL	Osterplant
AL	Parsnips
AL	Peppers (sweet)
AL	Rutabagas
AL	Sea lettuce
AL	Spinach
AL	Sprouts
AL	Swiss chard
AL	Watercress

Column No. 2
Proteins and Fruits

AC	Beef
AC	Chicken
AC	Cotage cheese
AC	Duck
AC	Fish
AL	Honey (pure)
AC	Lamb
AC	Mutton
AC	Oyster
AC	Rabbit
AC	Turkey
AC	Veal
AL	Apples
AL	Avocados
AL	Cranberries
AL	Dates
AL	Grapes
AL	Lemons
AL	Oranges
AL	Pears
AL	Pineapple
AL	Prunes
AL	Rhubarb
AC	Buttermilk
AC	Clams
AC	Crab
AC	Eggs
AC	Goose
AC	Jello
AC	Lobster
AC	Nuts
AC	Pork
AC	Raw sugar
AC	Turtle
AL	All berries
AL	Apricots
AL	Cantaloupes
AL	Curants
AL	Figs
AL	Grapefruit
AL	Limes
AL	Peaches
AL	Persimmons
AL	Plums
AL	Raisins
AL	Tomatoes

Column No. 3
Starchy Foods

AL	Bananas
AC	Beans (lima)
AC	Bread
AC	Chestnuts
AC	Corn meal
AC	Grapefruit
AC	Gluten flour
AC	Macaroni
AC	Millet rye
AC	Peanuts
AC	Peas (dried)
AL	Potatoes (white)
AC	Rice (brown)
AC	Roman meal
AC	Sauerkraut
AL	Squash (hubbard)
AC	Barley
AC	Beans (white)
AC	Cereals
AC	Corn
AC	Crackers
AC	Corn starch
AC	Lentils
AC	Maize
AC	Oatmeal
AC	Peanut butter
AC	Potatoes (sweet)
AL	Pumpkin
AC	Rice (polished)
AC	Rye flour
AC	Tapioca

8. COOKING

Cook with low heat, without water or with only a little water in waterless cookware, lid left on. Don't peek, leave lid on until done to avoid air exposure to hot food. Waterless cooking at 185 degrees destroys only 2% of nutrients, as compared to 20% in steaming (212 degrees) and 50% in boiling foods. Use unsprayed vegetables, if available, and prepare as soon after picking as possible.

9. BAKE, BROIL OR ROAST

If meat is used, choose lean meat, no fat, no pork. Never fry or cook in heated oils.

It is important for us to realize that we should take more of our foods on the raw side, which is not as fattening and which has the advantage of providing more live enzymes to help the body use its nutrients better. Raw vegetables in a salad are wonderful for us. We can even use raw asparagus, squash and spinach in salads.

We can put raw foods in a liquefier and have blended fruit or vegetable drinks. I call them *health cocktails.* Of course, we must be careful about adding cream or butter.

Most people eat too many acid-forming foods: *meat, eggs, milk, wheat products and starchy foods.* As we have mentioned, a government survey has shown that 54% of the average American diet is made up of wheat and milk products. These are the greatest weight builders when taken in excess. The American diet should only be 6% of these foods. We need to eat more fresh vegetables and fruits with our meals. In doing this, we reduce the taking of too many starches and proteins, and produce a better acid/alkaline balance.

Vegetables and fruits not only provide a vital source of vitamins and minerals, and a steady supply of glucose easily handled by the bloodstream, but they provide much needed fiber for colon health. A recent survey showed that 70% of Americans realized fiber is important; 30% stated that they obtained most of their fiber from meat, fish and dairy products. *The 30% were mistaken.* There is no fiber in these foods. Fiber is found in whole grain cereals and breads, fruits and vegetables. It can also be taken after meals in supplement form—1 teaspoon of wheat bran or psyllium husks. *SPROUTS OR RICE POLISHINGS ARE ALSO GOOD.* Fruit and vegetables, taken in the proportions recommended here, supply enough water that we don't need to drink as much.

As a rule, root vegetables are higher in calories than others. Remember this when planning meals.

The following instructions were given to the cooks at our sanitarium to carry out our idea of natural, whole and pure. These are not reducing ideas, but a maintenance diet for the average person. Most people will not gain weight on this diet. There are many lovely ideas here for those who want to get into food planning in the future.

Upon arising, drink a glass of warm water—add a teaspoon of liquid chlorophyll, if desired. This is especially effective as an aid to good bowel function.

One-half hour before breakfast, take unsweetened fruit juice such as grape, pineapple, prune, fig, apple or black cherry. Liquid chlorophyll in water or a broth or lecithin drink may be taken instead. Add 1 tablespoon vegetable broth powder and/or 1 tablespoon lecithin granules to a glass of warm water. Herbal teas are also recommended.

Between juice or drink and breakfast, I suggest that you skin brush for 2 to 5 minutes, exercise on a bouncer to music, take a walk in a garden or a short hike or do other exercise.

IN MY SANITARIUM WORK, I FOUND THAT THE AVERAGE PERSON TAKES TOO MUCH WHEAT AND MILK PRODUCTS. THESE ARE BUILT UP IN THE BODY OVER THE YEARS CAUSING CATARRHAL PROBLEMS. WHEN THESE CASES CAME IN, I CUT OUT ALL WHEAT AND MILK TO MAKE SURE THEY WERE DRAINED OUT OF EVERY TISSUE IN THE BODY. EVERY DOCTOR KNOWS THAT WHEAT AND MILK CAUSE FAR MORE CATARRHAL PROBLEMS AND ALLERGIES THAN ANY OTHER FOOD. I USE ONLY MILLET, RYE, BROWN RICE AND YELLOW CORNMEAL AS STARCHES. THESE SHOULD BE TAKEN IN CEREAL FORM ONLY. CUT OUT ALL BREADS, PIES, CAKES AND OTHER PASTRIES.

THE AMERICAN DIET IS MADE UP OF 29% WHEAT AND 25% MILK, WHICH IS 54% OF THE TOTAL DAILY AVERAGE DIET INTAKE. THIS IS A VERY POOR PROPORTION. DOCTORS ARE MAKING A LIVING ON THIS.

BREAKFAST IDEAS

Fresh fruit, health drink and 1 starch; or 2 fruits, 1 protein and health drink; or fruit only. In boiling water, soak dried fruits such as unsulphured apricots, prunes, figs, apples, pears for 5 minutes before using. Fresh fruit of any kind may be used—melons, grapes, peaches, pears, berries or baked apple. Use fruit in season when possible; don't eat melons and sour fruit together. Sprinkle baked or stewed fruit with ground nuts or nut butter, especially sesame nut butter.

The following menus are adapted from instructions to the kitchen staff members when my sanitarium at the Ranch was in full swing.

BREAKFAST

Fruit: One fresh fruit and one dried fruit. For reducing, cut down on dried fruits. Prunes have a lot of fiber.

Drinks: Milk, if desired. Whey. Tea—three different kinds of teas should be served during the day; five different kinds should be kept on hand in the kitchen.

Cereals: (Always serve five different kinds during the week.) Yellow cornmeal (twice a week). Muesli (twice a week). Rye, brown rice, millet. Whole grain cereal should be cooked over very low heat, tightly covered; use double boiler or soak overnight in boiling water in widemouth thermos.

Supplements: (For sprinkling on cereals or fruits) Wheat germ, rice polishings, flaxseed meal and sesame seed meal.

Eggs: Soft and hard boiled or poached.

Sunday Mornings: O.K. to serve cornmeal hot cakes (with honey or pure maple syrup).

Bread and Butter: Keep away from wheat.

Coffee Substitutes: Any of the toasted grain or vegetable-based products. 10 am. Juice time—vegetable or fruit; or substitute vegetable broth.

MONDAY
Fresh fruit
Reconstituted dried apricots
Millet
Supplements
Oatstraw tea
Add eggs or cottage cheese for protein

TUESDAY
Fresh figs
Cornmeal cereal
Supplements
Shavegrass tea
Add eggs or nut butter, if desired,
or raw applesauce and blackberries
Coddled egg, supplements, herb tea

WEDNESDAY
Fresh fruit
Reconstituted dried peacher
Millet cereal
Supplements
Add eggs or cheese for protein
Alfalfa tea

THURSDAY
Fresh fruit
Reconstituted prunes
Brown rice (cold or warm) with
raisins, cinnamon, sunflower seeds, honey
For protein, yogurt with fruit and nut butter
Supplements, herb tea

FRIDAY
Slices of fresh pineapple with shredded coconut
Buckwheat cereal
Supplements
Peppermint tea
or baked apple, persimmons, chopped raw almonds
Acidophilus milk, supplements, herb tea

SATURDAY
Muesli with bananas, dates and cream
Supplements
Dandelion coffee or herb tea

SUNDAY
Cooked applesauce with raisins
Rye cereal
Supplements
Shavegrass tea
or cantaloupe and strawberries
Cottage cheese
Supplements
Herb tea

TAKE A WALK!

Starting out with a new diet or eating regimen, it is best for the cook to allow the family a transition time to get used to the changes. Rushing people or trying to force them breeds counterproductive results. So, be patient.

The basics of this daily food regimen are two different fruits, six or more vegetables, one protein and one starch, using fruit or vegetable juices or herb teas as between-meal snacks. Chlorophyll tea (1 teaspoon liquid chlorophyll in cup of hot water) can be used in place of fruit juice. Use at least two green leafy vegetables every day. I advise that 50 to 60% of the total intake be raw food. Isn't that easy to remember?

Salad Bar: Olives, Waldorf salad (peel apples); once or twice a week. Gelatin mold (with shredded carrot and pineapple); once or twice a week. Stuffed celery (almond or cashew butter); twice a week. Dates, (almond or cashew butter); once a week. Stuffed dates (almond or cashew butter); once a week. Carrot and cashew salad (made with Champion juicer); once a week. Carrot and pea salad with cheese; once a week. Cole slaw; once a week.

Always Serve: Finely shredded carrots, beets, turnips. Carrot sticks, celery sticks, sliced tomatoes, sliced cucumbers, slice green peppers.

Anything Else in Season, used raw: Jicama, zucchini, summer squash, onions (small), parsley, watercress, endive.

Alfalfa Sprouts, served daily: Other sprouts, served occasionally.

Salad Dressings: Avocado, cheese and yogurt, nut butter, cottage cheese with blue cheese and yogurt, oil, vinegar and honey.

Vegetables: Two cooked. Use one grown under the ground and one grown above the ground. One bland vegetable must be served such as: beets, squash (yellow neck, banana, winter, etc.), zucchini, peas, carrots, string beans, wax beans, spinach, asparagus. Other vegetables may include a sulphur type (doesn't have to). They are: cabbage, cauliflower, brussels sprouts, onions, broccoli, turnips, kohlrabi. Steamed onions may be served (creamed with parsley; once a week, as a separate dish).

Starches: Brown rice (twice a week), baked potato (twice a week), lima beans, cornbread, yams.

Drinks: Milk, whey, buttermilk, nut milk drink (once a week), herb tea, coffee substitute.

SUGGESTED LUNCH MENUS

MONDAY
Vegetable salad
Baby lima beans
Baked potato
Spearmint tea

TUESDAY
Vegetable salad with health mayonnaise
Steamed asparagus
Very ripe bananas
or steamed unpolished brown rice
Vegetable broth or herb tea

WEDNESDAY
Raw salad plate w/sour cream dressing
Cooked green beans
Cornbread and/or baked hubbard squash
Sassafras tea

THURSDAY
Salad w/French dressing
Baked zucchini and okra
Corn on the cob
Rye Krisp
Buttermilk or herb tea

FRIDAY
Salad
Baked green peppers stuffed with eggplant and tomatoes
Baked potato and/or bran muffin
Carrot soup or herb tea

SATURDAY
Salad
Turnips and turnip greens
Baked yam
Catnip tea

SUNDAY
Salad w/lemon and olive oil dressing
Steamed whole barley
Cream of celery soup
Steamed chard
Herb tea

FOUR BEST STARCHES AND OTHERS

1. Yellow cornmeal; 2. rye; 3. brown rice; 4. millet; others; barley (winter starch); buckwheat, baked or dead ripe banana, winter squash, baked potato, baked sweet potato. For variety, include steel-cut oatmeal, whole wheat cereal, shredded wheat, rye crackers, bran muffins, bread (whole grain, rye, soy, cornbread, bran breads preferred).

BEST HEALTH DRINKS

Vegetable broth, soup, coffee substitutes, buttermilk, raw milk, goat milk, oat straw tea, alfalfa-mint tea, huckleberry tea, mint tea, whey, carrot juice, V-8 juice or any health drink.

VEGETARIANS

Use soybeans, lima beans, cottage cheese, sunflower seeds and other seeds; also seed butters, nut butters, nut milk drinks, tofu and eggs. Use meat substitutes or vegetarian proteins. Twice a week: Lo-fat cottage cheese or any cheese that breaks. Once a week: egg omelet. If you have a protein at this meal, health dessert is allowed, but not recommended. Avoid eating protein and starch together. They are deliberately separated on all meal plans so you will eat more vegetables. The noon meal may be exchanged for the evening meal, provided the same regimen is upheld. Exercise is necessary to handle raw food; generally more exercise is applied after the noon meal. Sandwiches, if eaten, should be combined with vegetables at the same meal.

DINNER

Protein: Meat (lean, no fat, no pork) such as: chicken, turkey, meatloaf, lamb roast. A meat meal is to be served three times a week.
Fish: (baked): ocean white fish, halibut, bass, trout, salmon loaf.

Fresh salmon and canned sardines are very high in RNA for tissue rebuilding. Have fish at least one day a week. Nut loaf for vegetarians. Cheese souffle', cottage cheese loaf, eggplant and cheese loaf.

Two cooked vegetables and salad, as for lunch.

Two nights a week: Fruit and cheese; assorted cheeses; Swiss, jack, cheddar, cottage cheese.

Yogurt: Assorted fresh fruits; three kinds, such as: melons, apples, persimmons, pears, cherries, berries, oranges, apricots, peaches, nuts and dates. Crackers: Rye-Krisp, Ak-Mak or sesame.

Juices: It is all right to have a juice in place of any meal. Those on juice diets should have juice every three hours, as follows: 8 am - fruit juice, 11 am - carrot juice, 2 pm - carrot juice, 5 pm - fruit juice.

SUGGESTED DINNER MENUS

MONDAY
Salad
Diced celery and carrots
Steamed spinach (waterless cooked)
Puffy omelet
Vegetable broth

TUESDAY
Salad
Cooked beet tops
Broiled steak or ground beef patties
Cauliflower
Comfrey tea

WEDNESDAY
Cottage cheese
Cheese sticks
Apples, peaches, grapes, nuts
Apple concentrate cocktail

THURSDAY
Salad
Steamed chard
Baked eggplant
Grilled liver and onions
Persimmon whip (optional)
Alfa-mint tea

FRIDAY
Salad w/yogurt and lemon dressing
Steamed mixed greens
Beets
Steamed fish (with lemon slices)
Leek soup

SATURDAY
Salad
Cooked string beans
Baked summer squash
Carrot and cheese loaf
Cream of lentil soup or lemongrass tea
Fresh peach gelatin
Almond nut cream

SUNDAY
Salad
Diced carrots and peas
Steamed tomato aspic
Roast leg of lamb
Mint tea

MENU EXCHANGES

If the noon and evening meals are exchanged, follow the same regimen. Starches make you sleepy; proteins are stimulating. If insomnia is a problem, the meals may be switched for better results. Starch meals are for physical labor; proteins for mental work.

Never eat when emotionally upset, chilled, overtired, overheated, ill or lacking the keenest desire for the simplest food. Missing a meal will do you more good. Some may want to have an extra juice about 8:00 pm.

Fruit juice may be: apple, grape, papaya or liquid chlorophyll (1/2 to 1 teaspoon to a glass of water). Liquid chlorophyll may be used at 8 pm instead of juice. Those trying to lose weight can substitute a chlorophyll and water drink for any fruit or fruit juice.

Desserts: Always allowed on Sunday and two times a week. Gelatin mold (two times a week). Homemade ice cream (frozen fruit, whey and honey). Carrot cake, custard, gelatin mold (cherry, grape, raspberry), Apple Betty or yogurt with fresh fruit.

Avoid: All fried foods, foods cooked in hot oil, salami, peanuts, peanut butter, sausage, pastry, chips, dips, chocolate and cream.

SUPPLEMENTS

Most people who have subsisted a number of years on poor diets find they are short of biochemical elements. They have lived on devitaminized, demineralized foodstuff. For this reason, we recommend several supplements for rebuilding and revitalizing. They are not necessary to the person who has been living correctly, not burning up chemical elements faster than they can be replaced, under normal circumstances and under the proper diet. These are needed to make up what we especially lack in the "average" American dietary habits.

Supplements should be used in the diet daily and served at the dining table. They help counteract the shortages found in the common diet today. Also add them to liquefied drinks, salads or even desserts.

Dulse. The highest source of iodine needed for proper thyroid gland function. (Most of my patients lack iodine.) Use 1/2 teaspoon daily.

Sunflower Seeds & Sesame Seeds. The vegetarian's best protein sources and a valuable gland and nerve food. Grind into a meal or nut butter.

Rice polishings. Very high in silicon—for skin and hair health, general vitality; the nerves and brain receive B-complex vitamins.

Wheat Germ. Vitamin B and vitamin E rich—heart and muscle vitamin. Use it raw and refrigerate for freshness.

Additional Supplements: Add sesame seed meal to the sunflower meal. Include flaxseed meal for bowel bulk and good elimination.

Use 1 teaspoon (heaping) of each supplement daily; add to cereal.

Flaxseed meal is a wonderful addition to the cereal bowl especially for children to keep their bowels regular. Flaxseed is also high in vitamins E and F. It is a bowel lubricant, regulator and bulk source.

Supplements don't have to be in pill form. A person has to be in good health to assimilate "pill" form supplements. The supplements just discussed can be assimilated by anyone, even though they are concentrated. Use them in cereals, tonics, drinks, dressings and almost any recipe. However, heat and baking destroy vitamin E and lecithin.

MORE HELPFUL FOOD AND MEALTIME TIPS

Because you are unique, there are most probably specific ways to enhance your weight loss program that will work very well for you but not necessarily as well for others. The reverse is also true. Don't get too excited when a friend "shares" some great new dieting or weight loss rumor from the grapevine at a family fitness center, aerobics class or health food store. *Be open-minded but be very cautious.*

One tip that has helped many people is to take four capsules or tablets of spirulina half an hour before mealtime. Another is to take a heaping teaspoon of bee pollen fifteen minutes before eating. Either one may reduce your appetite.

Apple cider vinegar and honey in a glass of water has helped some individuals lose weight. To 16 ounces of water, add 1 tablespoon of apple cider vinegar and half a teaspoon of honey. Take this morning and evening.

Limit your fat intake to what you get in foods such as avocado, eggs and nut butters. Be careful with salad dressings. Most are very high in calories.

Make sure you are getting enough iodine to keep your metabolism up and enough vitamin E. Use at least a half teaspoon of dulse flakes every day, or a dulse tablet with morning and evening meals. Under 40s, take 400 units of vitamin E per day, over 40s increase that to 800 units. If you are using wheat germ oil, you don't need the vitamin E. There is vitamin E in the wheat germ oil.

You may want to use niacin to flush the toxins from organs and peripheral tissues, to speed up the elimination process. Start with 100 mg at each meal and work up to 500 mg. From 100 mg to 500 mg, add 50 mg to the 100 mg every four days until you are finally having 500 mg. Niacin is vitain B-3, perfectly safe, but uncomfortable to some because of the release of histamines that cause the face, ears and neck to redden and tingle for 15 minutes to half an hour. The histaminic response is accompanied by a flushig of blood capillaries and increased circulation which may hasten the burning up of fat calories.

TAKE NOTICE

DR. JENSEN'S EXTREME HUNGER SNACK
(May Be Used In Place Of A Meal)

I call this my *Special Slim Shake,* and it can be used as a substitute for one or two meals each day, because it is such a great building food with only about half as many calories as a diet meal.

SPECIAL SLIM SHAKE RECIPE (185 Calories)

1 tbsp skim milk powder
1 tbsp honeybee pollen
1 tsp chlorella granules
   (or 6 tablets)
1 sliver avocado
   (or 1/2 banana)
1 glass apple juice
   (or 1-1/2 tbsp apple
   concentrate in glass
   of water)

Combine ingredients in blender and blend for 1 minute. Whey can be substituted for the skim milk powder to help develop the friendly bowel flora better. This formula builds the red blood cell count, keeps up the blood sugar level, supplies trace elements, provides amino acids, fatty acids and fiber, and is high in chlorophyll for cleansing the tissues.

8

What To Expect As You Improve

One of the wonderful advantages of my diet plan is that weight loss is accompanied by a gradual normalizing of the body chemistry as mineral and vitamin deficiencies are taken care of and as appropriate ratios of protein, carbohydrate and fat from high quality foods begin to change the body.

The human body is in constant change. Old cells die and new cells grow to take their places. Over a period of a year or so, most of the chemical elements of which we are made are replaced. We are physically renewed. Whether there is any improvement in this new body over the old one depends on you, what you have put in your mouth and what you have done with your body during that year.

The best attitude to develop is a positive expectation that proper nutrition and exercise are going to create the best body you could possibly have. You're going to feel better, enjoy yourself more, sleep better, have more energy, move more quickly and gracefully, and enjoy your work more. You will think more quickly and clearly. Begin to appreciate how your body feels. When you become sensitized to what makes your body and mind work better, you'll be more sensitive about what you put into them.

When you go through my diet plan and follow my *Health and Harmony Food Regimen*, your body will be replacing old tissue with better quality tissue. This will result in physical effects that the average person wouldn't experience on an average diet, but as you move to a better, more natural diet, you will move in the direction of better health.

118

Initially, you'll have less energy as the body adapts to its lower weight. Later, you'll have more energy, vitality and zest for life.

As your body is cleansed and renewed, you may experience disturbances that you don't understand or like. When heavy habitual use of coffee, tea, chocolate or cola drinks is stopped, headaches and depression may occur. This is because the removal of caffeine and other chemicals unnatural to the body creates a temporary imbalance in the blood chemistry which registers in the brain as a headache. *Usually the body is detoxified in three days and the symptoms vanish.*

Sometimes, however, our bodies, due to poor living habits and environmental pollutants, have accumulated more toxic substances and have developed more imbalances than we realize, **particularly when suppressant medications have been taken in response to colds, flu, hay fever, bronchitis, asthma, arthritis and other disturbances and diseases.** Fatty tissue, particularily, tends to store toxic debris and heavy metals. When toxic drug residues, old catarrh, heavy metals and other substances are released from tissue in the processes of cleansing and renewal, we may experience a temporary *healing crisis* which acts very much like disease conditions. Knowing what to expect will remove much of the anxiety at encountering these situations.

THE REVERSAL PROCESS

In contrast to current myths about *catching* diseases, most if not all chronic diseases are the natural result of unnatural lifestyle habits. We eat, drink, worry and think them into existence. We put junk food and alcohol into the fatigued body, then stay up till all hours "having a good time." We fight with our spouses, then go to bed with nerve acids and adrenaline eating us up. We work at stressful jobs day after day, pour down coffee, fight traffic on the freeway and watch the latest unpleasant news on TV—crime, war, disaster and so forth. All of this has its effects on the body—*negative effects.*

We come down with colds and flu, which are actually natural cleansing processes, and because we don't want the symptoms, we take powerful cold medications which suppress certain brain centers, stop the elimination of catarrh and toxic wastes, and block the body's natural ways of taking care of these things. Catarrh and toxins become locked into the tissue structure where they serve as more or less permanent irritants, degrading the surrounding tissue. Blocking natural cleansing processes like colds and flu sets up preconditions for more serious breakdowns and diseases later.

If we interrupt this pattern by shifting to a natural lifestyle, eating good food, exercising and taking care of our bodies, many things change inside the body. With the right nutrients available, body energies shift to assist internal organs in repairing themselves. We may feel tired and experience lowered vitality, but it is only tempory. Wonderful things are happening in the body. Our energy is being used for tissue rebuilding, so less of it is available for ordinary life tasks. But, it will return, with interest. This phase may last from ten days to two weeks.

Weight loss as developed in my program is a reversal process, reversing the accumulation of fatty tissue that contains toxic encumbrances. *Your health will improve as a result of it.*

As tissues in organ after organ are rebuilt, and long term vitamin and mineral deficiencies are taken care of, the metabolic level is increased. This, at some point, gives the tissues enough strength to start getting rid of some of those toxic wastes we have forced into them. This is usually a very rewarding weight loss period. There may be increased kidney and bowel elimination for a while before the body stabilizes.

It is especially important to take care of the urinary system during a time of elimination, and there are special foods, drinks, vitamins, minerals and herbs that help us cleanse and rejuvenate the kidneys, as shown in the following list.

URINARY SYSTEM

STRUCTURE: Kidneys, bladder, ureters, urethra.

FUNCTION: Elimination of liquid waste, regulation of chemical composition of blood, fluid and electrolyte balance and volume, maintenance of acid-base balance.

FOODS: Watermelon (including seeds), pomegranate, apples, asparagus, liquid chlorophyll, parsley, green leafy vegetables.

DRINKS: Celery/pomegranate juice; black currant juice/juniper berry tea; pomegranate juice/goat whey; celery/parsley/asparagus juice; beet juice; grapes; KB-11 tea; cleaver tea.

VITAMINS: A, B-Complex, B-2, B-6, C, D, E, choline, pantothenic acid.

MINERALS: Calcium, potassium, manganese, silicon, iron, chlorine, magnesium.

HERBS: Juniper berries, uva ursi, parsley, golden seal, slippery elm, elderflowers, ginger, dandelion, marshmallow.

The weight may stablilize or even increase for a time, but don't worry. More building and repair is going on inside the body at a faster rate. Even though you are on a lower calorie diet than before, your digestion and assimilation are so much better that food is more efficiently used.

THE HEALING CRISIS—A BLESSING TO BE WELCOMED

When you are feeling great, suddenly a healing crisis will erupt. If you have had boils or skin problems in the past, they may return. Colds, flu, fever, diarrhea—discharges from any or all orifices of the body may occur. The body is retracing its way back to health, and it stops at each point in the past where you have had some ailment or disease which was incompletely taken care of, and the same old symptoms return. Old stored toxic material is discharged. Again, this is a wonderful thing, although it can be most uncomfortable at the time. This is nature's way of healing, extremely thorough. **Don't try to stop it with medication.** It will stop itself in from three days to a week or so.

Symptoms experienced during the healing crisis depend on how well you have treated your body and on what ailments you have had in the past. The reversal process usually takes you from one ailment to another, (over a period of time) in reverse order of their appearance, so you experience the symptoms of the most recent ailment or disease first.

After the healing crisis, you'll feel great again. But that doesn't mean it's all over. You may go through several in the coming months and years, until all the old debris of past illnesses is cleaned out of your system. Once it is gone, it is permanetly gone and you do not have to experience any of those old troubles again if you are living right.

You may lose considerable weight during a healing crisis, but you will gain only part of it back. It may stabilize for ten days to two weeks after that, or you may continue losing weight as you stick to your diet.

KEEP TRACK OF YOUR PROGRESS

It is an excellent idea to see a doctor who knows nutrition before you start on a diet. It is a must if you are over 40 or over 10 pounds overweight, or if you have any chronic disease or physical condition that might be affected by diet and exercise changes. I believe that my reducing diet is safe to use with almost any state of health.

You may want to ask your doctor for the SMA Panel test to have some basis for checking your state of health and progress at suitable intervals.

TAKE A WALK!

9

Tips On Staying At The Right Weight

When you reach the weight that is natural for you, it will take fewer calories to keep you going than when you were overweight, with a few extra allowed to meet the needs of your exercise program. Weigh yourself once a week, and if you find your weight has crept up more than 3 pounds, *lose it*. You will know how by the time you finish this book.

Eat a wide variety of foods you like, based on my *Health and Harmony Food Regimen,* as presented in another chapter.

Remember, permanent lifestyle changes are the key to keeping slim and fit. These include changes in attitude, thinking, exercise, recreation, eating habits and anything else that has contributed to your gaining excess weight in the past. Buy new clothes that fit the new you, and enjoy the way you look and feel wearing them.

CHANGING FOOD HABITS

1. **Cut sugar and white flour products to a minimum.** Sugar drains vitamins from body reserves, throws calcium and the endocrine system out of balance and adds worthless calories to the diet. White flour, most of its food value removed during processing and bleaching, slows intestinal activities (which encourages weight gain) and is easily broken down to worthless sugar calories in the body.

2. **Cut down processed foods.** Their food value is reduced in

processing, and chemical additives in them may cause chemical imbalances or toxic reactions in the body.

POTASSIUM CONTENT IN FOODS
(Milligrams per 100 gram portion)

Molasses (blackstrap)	2927	Coconut, dry meat shredded	420
Yeast, torula	2046	Lamb chops, broiled	410
Yeast, bakers', dry, active	1998	Potatoes, boiled	407
Soy grits, low fat	1942	Broccoli, raw	388
Soy flour	1730	Kohlrabi, raw	382
Soybeans, dry, raw	1677	Bananas, ripe, raw	377
Apricots, dried	1561	Steak, rare	377
Lima beans, dry, raw	1499	Flour, wheat, whole meal	370
Rice bran, dry, raw	1495	Pasta, whole meal, dry	370
Peaches, dried	1191	Chicken, roasted	368
Wheat bran, dry, raw	1050	Currants, black, raw	360
Mung beans, dry, raw	1028	Squash, winter, boiled	360
Wheat germ, dry, raw	1020	Rolled oats, dry	354
Pistachio nut kernels, raw	972	Loquats, raw	348
Sunflower seed kernels, raw	920	Passionfruit, raw	348
Parsley, raw	903	Pumpkins, raw	340
Figs, dried	900	Peas, fresh, raw	338
Chestnuts, dried	875	Miso	334
Chestnuts, dried	875	Shallot bulbs, raw	334
Raisins, dried	840	Beet greens, boiled	332
Olives, green, fresh	809	Celery, raw	332
Chickpeas (garbanzos) dry, raw	797	Leeks, raw	330
Almond kernels, natural, raw	773	Radishes, raw	322
Lentils, brown, dry, raw	757	Beets, raw	320
Sesame seeds, whole raw	725	Leeks, boiled	320
Currants, dried	719	Nectarines, raw	307
Brazil nuts, raw	715	Carrots, raw	305
Hazelnuts, raw	704	Artichokes, globe, boiled	301
Peanuts, raw, without skins	700	Brussels sprouts, boiled	300
Spinach, raw	700	Watercress, raw	298
Prunes, dried	694	Apricots, raw	294
Cream cheese	686	Guavas, fresh	289
Dates, dry	648	Liver, raw	288
Spinach, boiled	637	Tomatoes, raw	287
Avocados, Fuerte	604	Cornmeal, dry	284
Pecan nut kernels, raw	603	Kohlrabi, boiled	278
Lima beans, boiled	602	Tuna, canned in water	275
Yams, boiled	590	Beans (long green), raw	272
Flounder, baked	587	Butternut squash, baked	271
Steak, well done	580	Cabbage, red, raw	268

Pears, dried	573	Broccoli, boiled	267
Beet greens, raw	570	Macadamia nuts, raw	264
Apples, dried	569	Cantaloupes	263
Parsnips, raw	541	Corn, sweet, raw	260
Soybeans, boiled	540	Pomegranates, raw	259
Garlic cloves, raw	529	Beans (long green), boiled	258
Parsnips, boiled	505	Cabbage, Chinese, raw	253
Potatoes, baked in skin	503	Cabbage, white, raw	250
Walnuts, raw	491	Chives, raw	250
Coconut, fresh meat	480	Turnips, raw	245
Mushrooms, raw	480	Tomatoes, boiled	244
Swiss chard, boiled	480	Sweet potatoes, raw or boiled	243
Broadbeans, fresh, raw	471	Maple sugar, pure	242
Rye, whole grain	467	Persimmons, raw	242
Cashew nut kernels, raw	464	Lentils, brown, boiled	240
Avocados, average	455	Pumpkins, boiled	240
Chestnuts, fresh	454	Turnips, boiled	240
Buckwheat, raw	448	Honeydew melons, raw	235
Salmon, baked	443	Okra, raw	235
Artichokes, globe, raw	430	Prune juice, canned	235
Millet, whole grain	430	Currants, red, raw	234
Artichokes, Jerusalem, raw	420	Papayas, raw	234

3. **Cut down salt or use a little evaporated sea salt instead.** Salt causes water retention and has been linked to hypertension and other diseases. Try herbs, broth powder and natural seasonings instead. *EAT ORE FOODS HIGH IN POTASSIUM, WHICH HELPS TO DRAIN THE WATER ACCUMULATION IN THE BODY.*

4. **Throw away the frying pan.** Avoid all fat-fried foods and foods cooked in hot grease or oil.

5. **Eat at mealtimes with your family.** You can eat what they do, only eat less than you used to eat. Always leave some food on the plate to train your mind to exercise discipline over appetite.

6. **Realize that feeling hungry does not mean you should immediately snack on something.** Hunger is a healthy feeling if restrained until mealtimes.

7. **Those who tend to hold water**—the hydripheric types—should eat high potassium foods often (see list under 3). Cleaver tea, KB-11 and

vitamin B-6 will help reduce water retention. It is also important to have adequate intake levels of vitamin B-12 and iron.

8. **Avoid fast food outlets.** Their food, as shown in surveys, is high in calories and salt.

9. **Cut down on fat-rich foods and alcoholic beverages.** Obvious sources of high-fat foods are whole milk, whole milk cheese, cream, butter, cream cheese, sour cream, fried foods, margarine, mayonnaise, many salad dressings, pork products (especially bacon), duck, ground meat, frankfurters and spare ribs. Not so obvious sources include avocados, chocolate, coconut, nuts and seeds.

10. **Plan ahead on how you will handle holiday meals at your home or with relatives.** You can simply control your eating, or you may wish to skip or skimp on aother meal or two so you can sonsume more at the holiday meal.

CHANGING YOUR BEHAVIOR

Unless your motivation and behavior are in line with your goals, the best diet plan in the world will do you no good. My diet plan is designed for mature adults who are willing to make the necessary changes in lifestyle to bring their weight down and keep it where it belongs. According to the research of Dr. Albert J Stunkard from the *University of Pennsylvania School of Medicine,* there are five basic steps to increase your chances of success in losing weight.

1. Keep daily records of what you eat and how much you exercise.

2. Watch out for places, events and times that stimulate a desire to snack, and change them as necessary. If you have always snacked before bedtime, for example, try doing a crossword puzzle or having a cup of herb tea instead. Don't try to simply suppress old habits; exchange them for better ones.

3. Change the way you eat, especially if you tend to gobble down food as you work or perform some other activity—such as reading or watching TV. When you eat, do nothing else but eat. Look at your food, savor it, enjoy each bite. Learn to be emotionally satisfied with it. When we rush through meals unconscious of our food, it is all too easy to overeat.

4. Reward yourself for successful weight loss or for maintaining a

healthy weight. Buy something you've wanted for a while, or go to the movies or a concert. It doesn't have to be a big thing. You can buy a little box of gold stars at a variety store and make up a score sheet where you give yourself a gold star each week for meeting your goals.

5. Be positive about your life changes. Avoid feeling sorry for yourself that you can't gorge on food any more, and concentrate on how much better you feel and look. *Avoid negative feelings about yourself and your weight.* Find good things to say and think. Take life a day at a time until you have maintained your natural weight steadily for six months.

We find that brain centers which seem to control habits may take months to adjust to a new lifestyle. This doesn't mean you will be tortured with hunger pangs during the intervening period, it only means you will have to exercise some prudence and caution.

If you are used to watching TV and drinking beer or eating peanuts when you come home from work, try taking a short nap or exercising instead. Get involved in more active things than you were before. Go roller-skating, see a baseball game or a ballet, take hikes, play tennis or racketball with a friend. Try to find some activity which helps lift others, and volunteer time for it.

The basic idea here is that sometimes food unconsciously becomes higher on our priority list of life events than it should be. When we stop and think about how much time, energy and money we put into food and food-related events, we may be very surprised, realizing that it is time to re-evaluate what is realy important in life. Then we can begin adding new activities and dropping old ones, to make changes in accordance with our new priorities.

10

Two Diet Plans For Losing Weight, Keeping Fit And Staying Healthy

In this chapter, I am going to present my Special Two Week Diet Plan and my 30-Day Diet Plan with two meal options, one for 1200 calories per day, the other for 1800 calories, each one nutritionally balanced. The fat content in both diets is sharply reduced since no fried or deep fat fried foods are allowed, and the use of fats and oils in meals is minimized. *The American average daily intake of fat is 40% to 45% of the diet, which the American Academy of Sciences tells us is double what we should be getting.* I have recommended a low-fat food regimen for over 50 years to my patients. You will get adequate amount of fats from the meat, fish, poultry, dairy products, nuts and seeds in my diet plan.

I recommend that physically active but overweight men and women (those who work at physically demanding jobs, who have a great deal of work to do at home or who exercise hard and regularly) try the 1800 calorie diet if they need to lose weight. Less active people should try the 1200 calorie diet.

People with chronic weight problems of many years standing should see a doctor, as we have mentioned previously that it could be an endocrine problem which needs more specialized assistance. *Those who always gain after dieting, especially when on a healthy way of living, need to seek out a nutritional counselor.*

Nutritional researchers recommend that women avoid diets under 1000 calories a day and that men avoid diets under 1500 calories, but both men and women whose lifestyle is more sedentary, more on the slow-and-easy side, will be all right on the 1200 calorie diet. If you are in doubt, check with your doctor and show him my diet plan. But, make sure he or

128

she knows something about nutrition so you'll be getting sound advice, not worthless opinion.

THE SECRET OF MY DIET PLAN

The secret of my diet plan lies as much in what is not in it as what is there. The primary benefit, I believe comes from two factors: *plenty of healthy fresh vegetables and fruits and reduction of fats, protein and refined carbohydrates.* You will notice there are no jams, jellies, pies, cakes, cola drinks or chips and dips in my diet plan. Refined white sugar, white flour products and most packaged, refined products are left out for reasons given in previous chapters. Pork is left out. Fatty meats and manufactured meat products like sausage and hot dogs are out. Butter is minimized. *WHOLE, PURE, NATURAL,* fresh foods are emphasized.

In an experiment, three groups of Swedish athletes were put on three different diets (high protein and fat, mixed diet, high complex carbohydrate diet) for three days, then given a bicycle-riding endurance test. The athletes on the complex carbohydrate diet, mostly fruit, vegetable, whole grain bread and cereal grains, outperformed the others by going three hours, as compared to two hours for the mixed diet group and one hour for the high protein group. My diet is also high in complex carbohydrates, *which means it is more sustaining than most other diets.*

You see, your body molds to what you put in it. Eating junk food builds a junk body. The body does its best with what you feed it, but the only way it can protest against wrong eating habits is by getting fatigued, sick, fat or unattractively thin. *That is something to stop and think about.*

Eating fresh, *WHOLE, NATURAL, PURE FOODS* builds a healthy, vitality-filled body. Now we find that people can overeat on healthy food just as they can on junk food. When comedian Dick Gregory first switched to a vegetarian diet, he thought he had to eat twice as much to make up for cutting out meat. Vegetarian foods can be very fattening if you don't know what you're doing. His weight soared to somewhere around the 300 pound mark, according to one magazine article. Then as he learned more about food and nutrition and began to eat properly, his weight dropped back to normal and he felt great.

Another secret of my diet plan is cutting back a little on protein, cutting back a lot on fats, increasing the complex carbohydrates and cutting out refined carbohydrates. There is plenty of fiber in my diet plan, lots of natural vitamins and minerals, and you will find variety and simplicity in the foods recommended.

DON'T BE FOOLED BY MYTHS

Don't be fooled by that old myth which says vegetables and meat without salt are drab, boring and tasteless. *Nothing could be farther from the truth, and you have some wonderful surprises in store.*

Go to your local health food store and see what they have in the way of natural vegetable and herbal seasonings. Some of these are absolutely wonderful, with a satisfying salty taste. Quick-sip, a product that tastes similar to soy sauce, can be used on meats and vegetables, and it is delicious on the starchy grains such as brown rice, millet, buckwheat and so forth. There is no salt in these preparations.

Don't try to cheat by using salt substitutes (I think they are worse than salt), lots of salted butter, or by using white rice and other quick-cooking substitutes for the natural grains in the diet plan. You'll only be cheating yourself of nutritional value and of the wonderful discoveries you'll be making by honestly trying to change eating habits. You can use a little sea salt--but go easy on it. Salt holds water in the body.

Now, I am not telling you that food will not taste different, even somewhat bland, when you first switch to your new diet. It will take a week or two for your taste buds to get rid of that burned-out quality due to heavy salt and spice use in the past. Then, what you eat will begin to taste wonderful.

WHAT ABOUT HERBS?

Many times I caution patients about spices and spicy foods, because they tend to be hard on the liver. Many spices irritate the gastrointestinal tract. The wonderful thing about herbs is that they not only enhance flavor but contain vitamins, minerals and other nutrient substances that contribute to better health. And, we find the great majority of them are extremely low in calories and are absolutely safe.

HERBS TO DELIGHT THE TASTE

Anise leaves, with a light, sweet licorice flavor, are very nice in salads, or on fish and poultry.

Basil, one of the most popular herbs used in cooking, is excellent in salads, soups, sauces, meats and stuffing. Use fresh leaves of Sweet Basil if available.

Bay leaves make a tasty addition to soups, stews and roasts.

Borage, a large flowering plant greatly loved by honeybees, has a light, cucumber-like taste. Use young leaves and flowers in salads.

Burnet is good in salads, similar in taste to borage. The chopped leaves are good in soups and sauces. The finest French dressings are flavored with Burnet.

Caraway leaves in vegetable, fish and meat dishes are very good; the seeds are sometimes used in bread.

Chervil, called the "gourmet's parsley," enhances the taste of other seasonings and has a unique flavor of its own. Use in soups, salads and sauces.

Chives are familiar to most, but if you haven't used them, try cutting them into soups, salads, sauces or onto any food whose taste would be enhanced by a mild onion flavor. Many people like chives on baked potato.

Corriander leaves, fresh, are not widely available outside the Southwest where many supermarkets carry them, but you can grow your own easily from seed. For a cool, distinctive flavor, try it on fish, in salads, soups, stews, sauces, vegetables and virtually any main dish.

Costmary or "Bible leaf" was put in books in days past to keep out silverfish. It is a nice herb for salads, teas, meat, poultry and fish chowder.

Dill leaves are good in tuna or chicken salad, while the seeds are sometimes used in bread, omelets, meat, poultry and herb butters.

Gotu Kola, familiar to many as an Oriental medicinal herb, makes a tasty salad green.

Lemon Grass makes a lovely tea, especially delicious as an ice tea on hot summer days.

Lemon Verbena, one of the most fragrant herbs, is a nice addition to fruit salads and fruit drinks.

Licorice Mint, strongly flavored, is good in fruit salads.

Marjoram is a standard seasoning herb from a small bush. Try it fresh in salads or with tomato slices or in soups, sauces, meat dishes and fish. Sweet marjoram is the best seasoning.

Mint leaves (fresh) are lovely in salads. Spearmint is a favorite seasoning for lamb.

Oregano is another of the very popular herbs *Almost any food flavor is enhanced with oregano.* Greek Oregano, new to many in this country, has a stronger flavor.

Parsley is a nice addition to soups, salads, sauces and omelets. It is loaded with vitamin A and other vitamins.

Rosemary is another popular herb. Just a sprig in soups, stews and sauces adds a nice flavor.

Sage creates a lovely savory taste when added to eggs, soups, fish, meat and stuffing. This is another well-known seasoning.

Savory, once called "poor man's pepper," adds zing to soups, sauces and salads. Use only a sprig or less until you've sampled the flavor. Summer Savory is preferred in salads, while Winter Savory is considered wonderful with green beans.

Sorrel (French) has a somewhat sour flavor and is nice in salads or cooked with spinach or chard.

Tarragon (French) is used to flavor vinegar. Fresh Tarragon has 10 times as much flavor as the dry.

Thyme, a small leaved plant with a marvelous fragrance, is used in salad dressings, stuffings, omelets, sauces and with meats and eggs. English Thyme is the most popular, while French Thyme is milder.

Watercress, a nice salad green, is surprisingly high in vitamins, minerals (especially potassium) and even protein. Potassium helps keep water absorption down in these who tend to hold too much water in their tissues.

Most of this information was adapted, with permission, from *"Herbs for Your Kitchen,"* a guide and herb catalog published by *Taylor's Herb Gardens, Inc., 1535 Lone Oak Road, Vista, CA 92083.* Herbs and seeds can be ordered from this nationally known and respected herb nursery.

I strongly encourage you to experiment with herbs in your cooked and fresh raw foods. It's a whole new lovely world, and you won't be disappointed.

VEGETARIAN DIETS AND HEALTH

Research has shown that vegetarians have lower blood levels of cholesterol and triglycerides than meat eaters. A vegetarian diet is not for everyone, but for those whose lifestyles and personal preferences permit it, vegetarianism may be the healthiest way to live—and the slimmest.

Let me pause for a word of caution. The reason I use the phrase *for those whose lifestyles and personal preferences permit it* is because there is more to vegetarianism than meets the eye. I do not believe vegetarianism is consistent with a high-stress job or lifestyle. I think it is difficult to be a vegetarian in a fast-paced, conflict-ridden environment. Vegetarianism requires a *peace and harmony* way of life, and if you are not prepared to live that way, you may not be ready to be a vegetarian. It is also unrealistic, if you have enjoyed and eaten meat for many years, to make an intellectual decision to suddenly switch to vegetables strictly for health reasons. I'm not saying it is impossible, but it is very difficult.

I must also warn that overeating vegetarian foods can lead to obesity just as overeating nonvegetarian foods does. The same principle applies. **If you take in more calories than you use every day, the excess calories will be stored as fat.**

LET'S HAVE A CLOSER LOOK AT VEGETARIANISM

According to an article in the **New York Times**, about 10 million Americans say they are vegetarians, while millions of others deliberately limit their use of meat and poultry. In the past, the main questions regarding vegetarianism were centered around whether you could get enough protein, vitamin B-12 and iron from such a diet. Many cases of deficiencies were found among vegetarians in decades past, but times have changed.

Enough is now known about nutrition to allow planning a diet that provides sufficient amounts of all nutrients, even for fast growing children.

A 20-year study of Seventh-day Adventists by Dr. Roland Phillips and Dr. David Snowden has turned up some interesting health facts. About half of this religious demonination is made up of lacto-ovo-vegetarians, which means they use eggs and milk products as well as vegetables, grains and fruits. The two doctors found that older men who ate meat six times a week or more were twice as likely to die of heart disease than older men who do not eat meat. Middle-aged meat eaters were four times as likely to die of heart attack than non-meat eaters in the same age group. (Women are protected from heart disease by their hormones until menopause.) Seventh-day Adventists have lower rates of cancer of the breast, ovaries, prostate and pancreas; they are half as likely to develop cancer of the colon or rectum. Only 15% of the vegetarian Adventists are overweight, compared to 30-40% of the meat eaters. In the American population as a whole, 60% are considered overweight. Strict vegetarians who do not eat eggs or milk products tend to be the leanest because they get less fat, more low-calorie vegetables and fiber.

Studies in Italy have shown that soy protein lowers blood cholesterol better than a low-fat, low-cholesterol diet. A study in Israel indicated a low 2% of vegetarians had high blood pressure, compared with 26% of non-vegetarians. Researchers from Australia found that when meat users changed to a vegetables, milk and eggs diet for six weeks. their blood pressure dropped. When they returned to their normal meat-eating routine, it went up again. A Boston study, in which eight ounces of meat was added daily to the diets of strict vegetarians, showed an increase in blood cholesterol of 19%.

We find a decisive lowering of cancer and heart disease among vegetarians, but there is some debate as to the true reason. Dr. Alex Hershaft points out that not only does meat contain saturated fat and cholesterol, but often pesticides, hormones and residual antibiotics from the cattle feed as well. Toxic substances like these are concentrated 20 times higher in the fatty tissue as in the meat. (One of the best reasons for reducing is that toxins and heavy metals are concentrated in human fat, too.) It is probable that the toxins in the animal fat, nonexistent before the 20th century, play a significant role in the genesis and growth of chronic disease in meat eaters.

What about getting enough protein from vegetarian foods? For one thing, the egg is the most efficiently matched protein to the needs of the human body. It has all the nutrients required to make life, including all eight amino acids essential to human nutrition. It is also possible, by combining certain vegetarian foods, to make a complete protein out of two foods deficient in one or more of the amino acids. These must be eaten at the same meal.

For example, bread is deficient in two essential amino acids, but if it is eaten with cheese, the combination is a much higher quality protein than either alone. Dairy products and grain products are, generally speaking, an excellent combined protein. Since Americans use so much milk and wheat in their daily diet, it is best to limit these in a vegetarian diet to avoid excess catarrh and possible allergies. Try to use other grains often and use wheat only once in a while. Milk and milk products also supply the amino acids that are deficient in seeds, nuts, beans and potatoes.

HIGHEST PROTEIN VEGETARIAN FOODS
(Percent of Food as Protein)

Soy grits, low-fat	47.3	Wheat bran	14.6
Gluten flour	41.4	Brazil nuts, raw	14.3*
Brewer's yeast	38.8	Creamed cottage cheese	13.3
Soy flour	38.6	Rice bran	13.3
Soy milk, dry	34.1	Whey powder	12.9
Pignolia nuts, raw	31.1	Hazelnuts, raw	12.6
Pumpkin seeds, raw	29.0	Eggs, whole	12.5
Swiss cheese	28.8	Rye, grain	12.1
Peanuts, raw	26.5	Rye, flour	11.9
Peanuts, roasted	26.4*	Buckwheat	11.7
Wheat germ	26.3	Wholewheat flour	11.5*
Sunflower seeds, raw	24.0	Pasta	11.5
Garbanzo beans	20.5	Soybeans, cooked	11.0*
Almonds, raw	19.5	White flour	11.0*
Pistachios, raw	19.3	Miso	10.5
Sesame seeds, raw	18.6	Wheat, whole grain	10.2*
Cottage cheese uncreamed	18.2	Millet, whole grain	9.9
Cashews, raw	17.2	Corn meal, dry	9.2
Ricotta cheese	16.7	Cream cheese	9.0*
Egg yolks	16.2	Cracked wheat bread	8.5*
Walnuts, raw	14.8	Boiled lima beans	8.2*

*High in fats or carbohydrates.

Legumes mainly lack the amino acid tryptophan and those amino acids containing sulphur. Tofu, which is soybean curd, is deficient only in the sulphur amino acids, (as are soybeans). Grains complement legumes almost perfectly. Good combinations include:

Soybeans, rice, wheat
Soybeans, peanuts, sesame seeds
Soybeans, wheat, sesame seeds

Soybeans, corn, milk
Legumes and rice
Beans and wheat
Beans and corn
Beans and milk
Rice and wheat

Vegetables tend to lack sulphur-containing amino acids, so to increase their protein value we could serve them with sesame seeds, millet, rice or mushrooms (all high in the sulphur amino acids). It is well, in general, for vegetarians to consider having bread, corn bread or a cereal grain with salads or other vegetable dishes to enhance protein value.

HOW FATTENING IS CHEESE?

When we look at how cheese is made, we find out that the whey is taken out and it is not a true "whole" food. Whey is high in natural sodium, wonderful for the digestive system and joints, but in cheese they replace this natural sodium with table salt sodium, which is not good for us.

I feel cheese is still one of our better proteins, considering the other proteins available to us, but we need to realize we have to be careful in selecting cheese, like any other food.

Because of the salt and saturated fats in cheese, we should know it is fattening if used too much. Cheese is a good cell-building, cell-repairing food, but it is not a perfect food, so we must be careful to use it in moderation.

A vegetarian reducing diet can be used just as easily as one containing meat, and it will reduce blood cholesterol and triglycerides more rapidly. Care must be taken to get sufficient protein, iron and vitamin B-12. Arrange meals so that each day the calorie count is at least 1000 calories for women, 1500 calories for men, with about 16% protein, 64% carbohydrates and 20% fat. Sufficient fat is generally available if eggs, whole grains, nuts and seeds are included each day. Most raw nuts and seeds are over 50% vegetable lipids, the healthiest kind, with no cholesterol.

FAT LEVELS IN CHEESE (GRAMS PER OUNCE)

Low Saturated Fat

Dry-curd cottage cheese	0.08
Low-fat cottage cheese 1%	0.18
Low-fat cottage cheese 2%	0.35
Creamed cottage cheese	0.81
Part skim ricotta	1.38

Moderate Saturated Fat

Whole milk ricotta	2.32
Part skim mozzarella	2.87
Low-moisture, part skim mozzarella	3.08
Mozzarella	3.73
American pasteurized process cheese spread	3.78

High Saturated Fat

Neufchatel	4.20
Feta	4.24
Camembert	4.33
American pasteurized process cheese food	4.38
Low-moisture mozzarella	4.41
Hard Parmesan	4.65
Port duSalut	4.73
Limburger	4.75
Tilsit	4.76
Provolone	4.84
Edam	4.98
Gouda	4.99
Swiss	5.04
Blue	5.30
Brick	5.32
Gruyere	5.36
Grated Parmesan	5.41
Muenster	5.42
Gjetost	5.43
Fontina	5.44
Roquefort	5.46
Pimento (pasteurized process)	5.57
American (pasteurized process)	5.58
Colby	5.73
Cheddar	5.98
Cream cheese	6.23

HIGH IRON FOODS
(Milligrams per 100 Grams)

Rice bran, dry	20.5	Soy grits	9.3
Brewer's yeast	17.3	Soy flour	7.4
Blackstrap molasses	16.1	Pistachio nuts	7.3
Pumpkin seeds	11.2	Sunflower seeds	7.1
Sesame seeds	10.5	Millet	6.8
Wheat germ	9.9	Parsley	6.5

HIGH B-12 FOODS
(Micrograms per 100 Grams—6 Micrograms Needed Per Day)

Cheese	1
Egg yolk	6
Kelp	N/A
Milk	N/A
Spirulina	200
Eggs, whole	2
Dried whey	2

Keep in mind that a vegetarian diet is not for everyone. Those who want to try this regimen might consider easing into it gradually. Just cutting out meat does not make a balanced vegetarian regimen. Vegetarianism is a mental discipline as well as a food regimen, and many vegetarians practice it for ethical or spiritual reasons. To many, vegetarian is associated with a philosophy of pacifism, or even peaceful coexistence with all life. It can take ten years for the body to adjust to a vegetarian diet, and there are some who will never be vegetarians because the lifestyle they have chosen is incompatible with vegetarianism.

VARIETY IS ESSENTIAL

One of the greatest things I can tell you about diet, health and nutrition is that a variety of good foods is essential. Variety will help you lose weight and stay at the weight you should be. Variety helps guarantee that the vitamins, minerals, enzymes, proteins, carbohydrates and lipids you need to feed the brain, nerves, glands, muscles, bones, teeth and vital organs will be sufficient to keep you fit and full of vitality. Variety reduces the need for supplementary vitamins and minerals and cuts down those occasional urges to binge on certain foods.

Too many people get into food ruts. Breakfast has to be bacon, fried eggs, hash browns, toast and coffee, or it just isn't breakfast. Lunch has to be a ham sandwich and potato chips. Dinner has to be meat, potatoes and dessert. If this is you, you don't know what you're missing—or what your body is missing. Not only are you missing out on a wonderful array of taste treats and delightful food adventures, but your body is most likely short of vital nutrients. I believe that strictly limited food patterns, together with lack of exercise, are responsible for most of the chronic diseases we find today. A few foods are over-represented at mealtimes while the body is starving for others.

Let's start thinking in terms of variety. Don't stick to the same ingredients in your salads all the time. Use different kinds of leaf lettuce, not your favorite all the time. Put some raw spinach leaves in, or dandelion greens or wild miner's lettuce. Put in bits of broccoli and cauliflower as well as the usual celery, onions and tomatoes. Make hearty vegetable soups with different vegetable combinations. Don't have orange juice every morning—try grape juice, apricot nectar, pineapple juice or a combination like apple-cherry juice. Use a different salad dressing every day.

Cooking can be fun, and mealtimes can become wonderful adventures. Every food has a unique taste to itself, something to discover and savor. Jump out of the food rut, if you're in one, and learn to have a good time with your meals.

SUPPLEMENTS AND COUNSELING

It is often helpful to take supplements when following a reducing diet, not only to avoid aggravating previously existing vitamin and mineral deficiencies during the period of lower daily calorie intake, but also to prevent complications from any condition you may have. For the latter reason, it is best to get counseling from a nutritionist before beginning a reducing diet.

Millions of Americans who carry undiagnosed hypertension, Type II diabetes, hypoglycemia, atherosclerosis, hypothyroidism, anemia and other conditions need qualified professional advice before dieting. Supportive supplements may include a good multiple vitamin-mineral tablet each day, natural laxatives, fiber, diuretics, heart support and glandular system support.

I have frequently found overweight patients at the Ranch to have an underactive thyroid, and it is very important for such persons to take a thyroid supplement to avoid further glandular imbalances. Check with your doctor first.

Potassium is particularly indicated as a supplement during reducing programs, to help protect the heart and to counter the water retention effect caused by excess sodium. Your doctor will be able to help select the supplements you need.

SUPPLEMENTS I RECOMMEND

I always recommend supplements which I know to be of help in reducing. Four alfalfa tablets should be taken at the beginning of each meal, cracked between the teeth and swallowed with water to promote bowel health and cleanliness. Two digestaids and one Pancreatin tablet can be taken with each meal to improve digestion and assimilation. One or two beet tablets with each meal aid liver function and serve as a mild laxative. Wheat bran or psyllium husks adds bulk and fiber to the bowel and speed up the elimination. Take a teaspoonful after each meal.

I recommend a tablespoon of wheat germ oil twice a day, a teaspoon of rice polishings three times daily and 50 mg of vitamin B-3 after every meal. KB-11 or Cleaver tea, available at most health food stores, can be taken between meals to stimulate the kidneys. If the kidneys become overworked, I advise patients to cut down on fruit and fruit juices, especially citrus. Liquid chlorophyll in a glass of water is a wonderful cleansing drink which has no calories whatsoever. If water retention is a problem for you, use herbal extracts or tablets instead of teas and chlorophyll drinks.

DO YOU KNOW HOW TO EAT?

Everyone knows how to stuff food in his mouth. But, I have found many people who do not know how to eat. Does that surprise you? Eating is considered an art in some places, but I am talking about something a little different. For proper digestion and assimilation, we need to know how to eat properly.

These are those who bolt down their food, like starving wolves. There are parents who wait until dinnertime to criticize or discipline their children. There are husbands and wives who argue at mealtimes. There are those who read a book or newspaper while they eat, hardly aware of whether they are consuming food or their napkin. And, last but not least, there is the TV dinner crowd. I don't mean those who eat prepackaged TV dinners, but those who sit and eat while absorbed in their favorite soap opera, sports event or series program. Both reading and TV watching involve the functioning of the nervous system and glands in ways that can interfere with digestion and assimilation.

Keeping at the right weight isn't a matter of always eating the low-calorie foods, it's often a matter of eating only when we are truly hungry. We don't have to eat just to keep our stomach full. Some people believe that three meals a day are absolutely necessary, and I think in most cases we find out that to miss an occasional meal or to have a very small meal could be very good for us.

It is more important to eat only until our hunger is satisfied than to see how much we can eat. When we overeat we abuse the digestive system. If we don't have enough, we starve. We can starve for a short time and live on accumulated fat, protein and starch reserves in the body, but we find out there is a limit to our reserves. That's why diets are not the best for us.

Mealtimes should be special, pleasant occasions when the whole family gets together to do nothing else but eat and enjoy one another's company. Talking is fine, but it must be limited to positive, enjoyable subjects. If a child talks so much that his or her food is getting cold, the parents, of course, should lovingly insist that the child eat and save some of the conversation for later.

Pay attention to the food, right from the start. If you are a man, compliment "the cook" often for her work and artful preparation. Notice dishes that look especially attractive or that have a wonderful smell, and remark about them out loud. When you try your first few bites, tell the others how good you think the food is. Look at what you are eating; notice the color, texture and savory scent of it; savor it in your mouth. Chew well and slowly. If you are in the habit of rushing, put your fork down between bites until each mouthful is thoroughly chewed.

If you are "the cook," I want to encourage you to make the food served look nice as well as taste nice. Beauty is a wonderful aid to the digestion. When you come to the table yourself after preparing a lovely meal, don't hesitate to say things like, "Doesn't this look nice?" or "M-m-m-m, everything smells wonderful!" Feel free to do this whether anyone else says anything or not. Cooking is a special art and skill, and you have every right to feel proud or your cooking—and to enjoy it with relish.

I make these suggestions not to encourage meaningless rituals, but to stir the digestive juices, to stimulate the brain and nerves to prepare the digestive system to function efficiently. When we both enjoy and pay attention to our food as we eat, I believe digestion and assimilation are more efficient. We get more nourishment from our food—and there is less chance of overeating. When we eat too fast, our brain doesn't get the signal to stop eating until we have overeaten, and this is a common experience for many chronic overweight persons.

Reading or watching TV at mealtimes reduces stimulation of the gastric juices and sometimes places the glandular system in opposition to the digestive system. If what you are reading or watching is exciting, adrenaline is released from the adrenal glands, which causes constriction of the blood vessels to the stomach and bowel, hindering digestion and assimilation. My advice is, **don't do it**. You're wasting food, money and putting a strain on your digestive system.

It is especially important for those watching their weight to never eat a heavy meal later than 2 hours before bedtime.

COOKING TIPS TO GET MORE FOR YOUR MONEY

One of the most frequent wastes of food budget money and nutrients is to overcook food, destroying vitamins, enzymes and minerals. A friend of mine who visited South Africa commented on the high incidence of hardening of the arteries and relatively poor health among urbanized natives. Blacks who live in the rural villages of South Africa are often very healthy on a diet high in whole grain cereals and vegetables, with a little meat now and then. But when they move to the cities, many subsist on a sort of stew made by boiling water, vegetables, meat and as much as a handful of salt, together. After the solids are eaten, the leftover liquid is thrown away, along with whatever vitamins and minerals have not been destroyed by the prolonged cooking or exposure to air during cooking. *This is a disease diet, for the body can't long subsist on overcooked, depleted, devitaminized foods.*

The best way to cook almost anything is at low heat until just barely done. For fruits, this means when they are soft. Vegetables should still have an edge of crispness to them and possibly be a little underdone. Meat should be baked or roasted in the oven at low heat over as long a period of time as is possible without undue inconvenience. Cookbooks like those of the late Adelle Davis give instructions for doing this. Most juices and flavor are retained.

I believe the best way to cook vegetables is in low heat, waterless, stainless steel cookware. Second best is steaming them. Many stores now carry stainless steel steamer inserts, short-legged, round, folding-leaved devices that fit inside pots to keep vegetables, grains or other foods above the water as they cook in the steam. Electric crockpots are all right, and using a pressure cooker now and then is acceptable. However, I do not believe microwave oven cooking is necessarily wise, because we don't fully understand what effects can come from using intense radiation to cook foods.

When you go to the supermarket, you usually try to make the most of your food dollars. Don't throw them away later by overcooking.

A good tip—save the vegetable water when you steam vegetables and use it to make soups or to cook whole grain cereals. That cooking water has good vitamins, minerals and flavor in it, and adds to the taste of anything you use it with.

GETTING DOWN TO BUSINESS

Now it is time to talk business about starting your diet. We find it is always best to think and plan ahead, to make sure everything goes smoothly.

Your family can eat everything you will be eating, the only difference being that they will be able to eat more of some things than you are allowing yourself. If my diet is extremely different from your former family food pattern, you may have to ease them into it. For example, if they are used to eating a good deal of pork and beef, gradualy cut down on the number of times per week they are served. Use more chicken and fish. Encourage them to eat more vegetables. Their health and vitality will improve, sometimes dramatically.

One of the most effective ways to lose weight by dieting is to "pair up" with at least one other friend and do it together. If your spouse needs to diet and is willing, that will be a big boost to both of you. Resolve in advance to encourage and compliment one another on looks and progress. Go shopping together and buy yourselves outfits in a smaller size than you wear now. Then, hang them up someplace in the house where you will see them often.

When going out to dinner, either at a friend's house or at a restaurant, eat a salad first at home to reduce any temptation to eat excessively or to make wrong food choices. It's much easier to avoid making inappropriate food choices once you've taken the edge off your appetite.

Remember, too, that a half-hour of active exercise each day, to the point of perspiring and breathing heavily, will raise your metabolic level for hours longer, helping burn off fat calories long after you have stopped exercising.

Think positively about yourself and your diet. Think positively about getting off the diet and onto a healthy way of living and eating, as described in a previous chapter. *Use your head to get ahead.*

Study my food charts and diet plan. Vegetarians can substitute dairy products, tofu, grains, legumes, nut and seed butters and eggs for meat. Nonvegetarians and vegetarians alike can make alterations as desired in meal composition, as long as the basic plan is followed. My food charts make it easy for you to rearrange any meal to suit your taste.

Water, herb tea, coffee substitutes, broth or vegetable juice may be taken between meals, *always at least an hour and a half before the next meal.*

Use a variety of salad dressings. I don't believe in using much oil on salads, since we get enough in other foods. You are allowed to use bleu cheese, roquefort, vinegar and oil, yogurt, avocado dressing, oil with lemon and honey and similar dressings.

SPECIAL NOTES ON SALADS

Salads are a key factor in any good weight-loss diet program, and it is possible to be very creative with them. A high-fiber diet helps drive excess cholesterol out of the system, tones the bowel and ensures regularity. Best vegetables for salads are the leaf lettuces (head lettuce is almost nutritionally worthless), spinach leaves, watercress, parsley, celery, cucumbers, tomatoes, alfalfa sprouts (and other sprouts), onions, garlic and grated raw vegetables such as carrots, beets, parsnips, zucchini, turnips and so on (only use a little of each grated vegetable per salad and use 2 or 3). Some can't take the onions or garlic, or they live or work with people who can't take the odors, so use them with discretion.

There are many other things we can use in salads, such as avocado, sliced mushrooms, sliced raw green beans, raw pieces of cauliflower and broccoli, sliced bell peppers, chives, fresh corriander, herbs of various kinds such as anise, chard, miner's lettuce and raw beet, mustard, dandelion and turnip greens (these can become tough, so test first). Some things I don't believe in are croutons, bacon bits and other embellishments that usually come from packages.

It is a wonderful idea to mix or sprinkle wheat germ, which is high in magnesium, a little dulse flakes, grated cheddar or parmesan cheese, ground nuts or seeds in salads.

EXTREME DIETS

In extreme cases, I have used a special diet that is more effective in bringing weight loss, but it should only be used in consultation with or under supervision from a doctor. There are some persons who find it very difficult to lose weight on even a properly balanced reducing diet, and I have made a special effort to help them.

Some researchers have called the left side of the body the **negative** side and the right side, the **positive** side. Foods that feed the left side are called negative foods, such as potatoes, cereal grains, starches, sweet fruits and so forth; foods that feed the right side are called positive foods, such as meat, fish eggs, cheese, milk and so forth. Vegetables are neutral and can be used on both diets. **We never use citrus fruit with heart patients.**

The following is a right side or positive diet and should only be used *for three days to one week at a time, it should never be used by those with heart problems.* Most overweight people have taken too much of the starchy foods (I believe that people with heart disease need carbohydrates and starches in their daily food intake) in the past and that's why we give the more positive diet, to restore balance. Then we are ready to go on with my regular *Health and Harmony Food Regimen.* Understand that these extreme diets are only to be used for a limited time when a body is obese due to chemical imbalance. The following is an extreme positive diet and is only for balancing the body which is already in an extreme imbalanced direction.

Two or three meals per day, each to include:

Lean meat or fish
Sliced fresh tomatoes
One or two vegetables

Fruit with cottage cheese may be taken for breakfast. This diet burns fat rapidly but may cause heart palpitations, chest pains and other symptoms because this **positive** diet does not support the heart properly, which is on the left or **negative** side of the body.

In other cases, with people who had become overweight due to an extreme diet discrepancies I have used an extreme negative diet made up of:

Sweet fruits
Rice as a cereal and other starches
Low-calorie vegetables

This diet, too, must only be used under a doctor's supervision, because it is considered an extreme negative diet. This will support the heart well in many cases, but it is not a balanced diet. When this diet is over, it is best to start my *Health and Harmony Diet.*

TABLE OF FATTY FOODS TO REDUCE OR AVOID

FOOD	TOTAL FAT %	SATURATED FATTY ACIDS %	CHOLESTEROL (Mg/100 gm)
Lard	100	38	95
Oils:			
cottonseed	100	25	0
corn	100	10	0
olive	100	11	0
safflower	100	8	0
sesame	100	15	0
sunflower seed	100	12	0
Butter	81	46	250
Margarine	81	18	N/A
Pecans (raw)	71	5	0
Brazil nuts (raw)	67	13	0
Walnuts (raw)	64	4	0
Coconut (dried)	63	54	0
Hazelnuts (raw)	62	3	0
Bacon, fried	59	19	N/A
Almonds (raw)	54	4	0
Pistachios (raw)	54	3	0
Eggs, yolk only	31	10	1500
whole	12	4	550
Liver, average	4	2	300
Pork chops, broiled	38	14	70
Lamb chops, broiled	31	17	70
Veal chops, broiled	11	6	90
Cheese: Cheddar	33	18	100
Cream	32	18	120

LOWEST CALORIE VEGETABLES

The lowest calorie vegetable dish is a mixed green salad, two cups of which come to 50 calories or less. There are more than 50 calories in a tablespoon of dressing, so be conservative with the dressing. The following vegetables are cooked unless noted as raw; also see the Vegetable Chart later in the chapter. You can eat as much of these as you wish, especially the salad vegetables noted with an asterisk.

LOWEST CALORIE VEGETABLES

FOOD	AMOUNT	CALORIES
Fresh green string beans	1/2 cup	15
Beet greens	1/2 cup	9
Broccoli	1/2 cup	20
raw	1/2 cup	27
Cabbage (raw)	1/2 cup	12
Carrots	1/2 cup	24
Cauliflower	1/2 cup	10
raw	1/2 cup	15
Celery	1/2 cup	8
raw	1/2 cup	6
Cucumbers	10 slices	10
Garlic	1 clove	6
Eggplant	1/2 cup	17
Kale	1/2 cup	16
Leaf lettuce	1 cup	16
Okra	1/2 cup	11
Parsley	1/2 cup	13
Green peppers (raw)	1 medium	10
Radishes (raw)	1 radish	1
Summer squash	1/2 cup	12-17

TAKE A WALK!

TWO 30-DAY DIET PLANS

The two 30-day diet plans presented on the following pages are designed for you to create meals from calorie charts of the various food groups and foods I recommend. Meal planning and food selection are left up to you, so you can design meals uniquely suited to you (and your family, if you choose to include them). You may continue this diet for 30 days or as much longer as you desire, based on how you feel in body and mind. Consult your doctor if you feel you need professional advice.

1200 CALORIES/DAY DIET PLAN

BREAKFAST

HOW TO MAKE BREAKFAST

Our basic goal here is 2 fruits (or 1 fruit and 1 fruit juice) and 1 different cereal grain (no wheat) each day for 3-5 days before having the same one again. If you select 2 fruits, have a cup of broth, herb tea or chlorophyll and water half an hour before breakfast. *Count calories before preparing meal, staying as close as possible to 300. (If you plan to have a Waldorf salad, gelatin with fruit or mixed fruit salad for lunch, skip the breakfast fruit and add a selection from the Crackers and Bread Chart or Raw Nuts and Seeds Chart.)*

BREAKFAST—OPTION A—300 CALORIES
1 selection from the Drink Group Chart
1 or 2 selections from the Fruit Group Chart
1 selection from the Dairy Products Chart, Column 2, or
2 selections from Column 1

BREAKFAST—OPTION B—300 CALORIES
1 selection from the Drink Group Chart
1 or 2 selections from the Fruit Group Chart
Selection from the Cereal Grain Chart, Column 2, (no wheat)
1 selection from Natural Sweeteners Chart, Column 2

Notice that my Food Charts are varied enough to select too many calories or too few. If you are under 300 calories, fill in by adding a Ry-Krisp cracker or sprinkle a teaspoon of ground-up nuts or seeds on something you're eating.

SNACK—10 AM

Select 70-80 calories in one or more items from the Snack Chart. If you choose 80 calories in morning snacks, *I suggest you limit yourself to 60 or 70 in the afternoon.*

1200 CALORIES—LUNCH

HOW TO FIX LUNCH

Our basic goial here is to have 1 high calorie starch or 2 (1 high calorie, 1 low calorie starch)(such as baked potato, sweet potato, yam, brown rice, millet, squash and so forth, plus a variety of fresh raw and cooked vegetables. But if you had a Column 2 helping of a whole grain cereal (no wheat) for breakfast, you should have a protein at this meal. If you did not have fruit or fruit juice for breakfast, have a fruit salad for lunch.

LUNCH—OPTION A—400 CALORIES
1 selection from the Soup Chart
1 selection from the Salad Chart
1 selection from Salad Dressings (2 Tablespoons)
1 selection from Crackers and Bread Chart (no wheat)
1 selection from Cereal Grain and Starch Chart, Column 2
1 selection from Cereal Grain and Starch Chart, Column 2 (no wheat)
OR
1 selection from the Dairy Group Chart
3 selections from the Vegetable Chart

LUNCH OPTION B—400 CALORIES
1 selection from the Salad Chart
1 selection from the Cereal Grain and Starch Chart, Column 2 (no wheat)
OR
1 selection from the Dairy Group Chart
3 or more selections from the Vegetable Chart

150

You may use a little butter or margarine on your vegetables and, if you must have salt, use a little sea salt. Be sure to try one or more of the vegetable seasonings or broth powders available at your local health food store. They taste salty and add much more flavor than salt. You would be doing a favor to your body by switching from salt to a vegetable seasoning.

SNACK—3 PM

Select one or more foods from the Snack Chart, adding up to 60-80 calories. If you had an 80-calorie snack in the morning, don't go over 70 calories now. Save 50 calories for your evening snack.

1200 CALORIES—DINNER

HOW TO PREPARE DINNER

For the dinner meal, we always have a large vegetable salad and at least two cooked vegetables. Because many people prefer to have their main meat dish at this meal, I have put it here, but it is just as valid to have it at the lunch meal and have the main starch of the day at dinner. You can do this if you wish. Limit meat to one or at most two meals per week. Have fish or poultry at other times. An omelet or serving of cottage cheese occasionally is permitted.

DINNER—OPTION A—300 CALORIES
Large Salad of mixed raw vegetables
1 selection from the Meat, Poultry and Fish Chart
3 or more selections from the Vegetable Chart,
including 1 summer or winter squash

There is no second option for dinner, excepting the switching of the main starch to this meal.

AFTER DINNER SNACK
Choose any 50 calorie snack from Snack Chart.

1800 CALORIES/DAY DIET PLAN

The strategies for breakfast, lunch and dinner are no different on this diet as compared to the 1200 Calories/Day Diet Plan. The key is still to use whole cereal grains (no wheat), 2 fresh fruits daily, at least 6 vegetables, 1 starch and 1 protein. Keep in mind that 50-60% of the fruit and vegetables should be raw. Try to have a large mixed vegetable salad twice a day most days, and use the other salads for an occasional break in routine. I advise fruit salad no more than once a week. Remember, vegetables taste wonderful seasoned with some of the natural salt-free seasonings found in health food stores. There is no reason for your meals to be bland in taste. Learn to use herbal seasonings. *Add up calories before preparing meals.*

BREAKFAST—450 CALORIES
1 selection from the Drink Chart 1/2 hour before eating
(Take 1 fruit juice.)
1 selection from the Dairy Group Chart, Column 2
OR 2 selections from Column 1
1 selection from the Cereal Grain and Starch Chart (no wheat),
Column 1
2 selections from the Fruit Chart
1 selection from the Natural Sweeteners Chart

SNACK—10 AM
Select snacks totaling 100 calories from the Snack Chart.

LUNCH—600 CALORIES
1 selection from the Soup Chart (80 calories or more)
1 selection from the Salad Chart (double dressing okay)
1 selection from Column 1 of Raw Nuts and Seeds Chart
(add on salad)
1 selection from Column 2 of Cereal Grain and Starch Chart,
(no wheat)
1 selection from Crackers and Bread Chart (no wheat)

SNACK—3 PM
Select snacks totaling 100 calories from the Snack Chart.

DINNER—450 CALORIES
1 selection from Column 2 of Meat, Poultry and Fish Chart
1 large mixed vegetable salad with double dressing
4 selections from the Vegetable Chart, including 1 cooked green
vegetable, 1 root vegetable and 1 yellow vegetable and 1 squash
in season
1 selection from Crackers and Bread Chart (no wheat),
butter allowed

AFTER DINNER SNACK
Select snacks totaling 100 calories from the Snack Chart.

CEREAL GRAIN AND STARCH CHART

FOOD (COOKED)	COLUMN 1 AMOUNT	COLUMN 1 CALORIES	COLUMN 2 AMOUNT	COLUMN 2 CALORIES
Whole or cracked wheat	1/3 cup	70	--	--
Buckwheat groats	1/3 cup	60	--	--
Brown rice	1/3 cup	60	2/3 cup	120
Rolled or steel-cut oats	1/2 cup	65	--	--
Pearled barley	1/4 cup	72	1/2 cup	144
Whole or cracked rye	1/4 cup	67	--	--
Millet	1/2 cup	87	3/4 cup	130
Yellow cornmeal	1/2 cup	58	--	--
Yellow corn grits	1/2 cup	62	--	--
Cornbread	1 oz	55	--	--
Sweet potato	--	--	1 med (4 oz)	154
Baked potato	--	--	1 med (4 oz)	102
Lentils	--	--	1 cup	122
Yam	--	--	1 med (5 oz)	155

NOTE: Prepare millet and buckwheat by allowing 3 parts water to 1 part
grain; soak overnight in boiling water in widemouth thermos. Other grains allow
2 to 1. Always stir cornmeal or corn grits into cold water and bring to boil before
allowing to sit, to avoid lumping. Yams, sweet potatoes and potatoes can be
baked in the oven wrapped in foil to preserve moisture.

CRACKERS AND BREAD CHART

	AMOUNT	CALORIES
Ry-Krisp	2	60
Sesame	6	60
Ak-Mak	4	60
Rye bread	1 slice	56
Cracked wheat	1 slice	60
Whole-wheat	1 slice	55

(Pat of butter or margarine, 50 calories.)

NOTE: I am not in favor of including bread in diets, especially wheat bread, but if you must have it, here are the best breads to use. Avoid white bread. If you use butter or margarine, cut back those calories somewhere else.

DAIRY GROUP CHART

	COLUMN 1		COLUMN 2	
	AMOUNT	CALORIES	AMOUNT	CALORIES
Nonfat milk	1 cup	90	2 cups	180
Raw whole cow milk	1/2 cup	80	1 cup	160
Raw whole goat milk	1/2 cup	82	1 cup	164
Yogurt, plain	1/2 cup	80	1 cup	160
Low-fat cottage cheese	2/3 cup	80	1-1/3 cup	160
Egg, poached or boiled	1	80	2	160
Cream cheese	1-1/2 T	80	3 T	160
Bleu or roquefort	1-1/2 T	80	3 T	160
Cheddar cheese	1 oz	112	1-1/2 oz	168
Swiss cheese	1 oz	104	1-1/2 oz	156
Tofu	2/3 cup	80	1-1/3 cup	160
Ricotta cheese	2 oz	60	4 oz	120

SPECIAL NOTE: I have previously mentioned that the average American, in his daily diet, uses 25% milk and milk products, which is far too much. However, I do recommend yogurt and cheese, because they are among the best proteins I know. I *allow* milk but *DO NOT RECOMMEND IT.*

DRINK CHART

	AMOUNT	CALORIES
Apple juice	4 oz (1/2 cup)	63
Apricot nectar	4 oz	70
Grape juice	4 oz	80
Pineapple	4 oz	60
Prune	4 oz	85
Strawberry	4 oz	52
Cherry concentrate	1 tsp in 8 oz water	19
Vegetable broth	1 tsp in 8 oz water	3
Chlorophyll drink	1 tsp in 8 oz water	0
Lemon grass tea	8 oz	0
Comfrey tea	8 oz	0
Peppermint tea	8 oz	0
Shavegrass tea	8 oz	0
Spearmint tea	8 oz	0
Coffee substitute	8 oz	2

NOTE: Juices may be mixed half and half with cold herb teas to reduce the calorie intake or to extend the quantity while holding the calories constant. There is no caffeine in herb teas, and many of them have minerals needed by the body. They can be used as often as desired but should not be taken within half hour of meal times. Juices can also be mixed for delightful flavor surprises.

DRIED FRUIT
(3-1/2 ounce serving)

	CALORIES
Apples	289
Apricots	265
Banana	340
Currants	273
Dates	274
Figs	270
Pears	270
Peaches	263
Prunes	255
Raisins	279

NOTE: Dried fruit has more concentrated fruit sugars than fresh fruit because it has less water. Use them sparingly to sweeten other foods or reconstitute them (for winter fruits) by soaking them in boiling water.

FRUIT CHART
(Raw unless noted otherwise)

	AMOUNT	CALORIES
Apple	1 large	120
Apricots	2 medium	54
Avocado	1 large	360
Banana	1 medium	128
Blackberries	1 cup	46
Blueberries	1 cup	96
Cantaloupe	1/2 medium	40
Cherries	1-1/2 dozen	67
Cranberries	1 cup	48
Currants:		
red	1/2 cup	24
black	1/2 cup	30
Figs	1 med	30
Grapefruit	1/2 med	54
Grapes	1 cup	104
Guava (peeled)	1 medium	56
Honeydew melon	1/6 large	68
Loganberries	1 cup	64
Loquats	3-1/2 ounce	56
Lychees	3-1/2 ounce	64
Mango	1/2 medium	69
Muskmelon	1/2 medium	52
Nectarines	1 medium	50
Orange	1 medium	88
Papaya	1 large	160
Passion fruit	3-1/2 ounce	91
Peaches	1 medium	43
Pears	1 medium	111
Persimmons	1 medium	96
Pineapple	1 cup	73
Plums	2 medium	60
Prunes (cooked)	1 medium	43
Quince (cooked)	1 medium	51
Raspberries:		
red	1 cup	76
black	1 cup	91
Rhubarb (cooked)	1/2 cup	190
Strawberries	1 cup	55
Tangerines	1 large	52
Watermelon	8 oz slice	120

NOTE: You may want to use fruits as desserts or to sweeten other foods, such as cereal grains or plain yogurt. Use sun-ripened fruits where possible and avoid unripe fruits or fruits picked green for shipping to market. Fruits have more vitamins, vegetables have more minerals, generally speaking.

MEAT, POULTRY AND FISH CHART

	COLUMN 1		COLUMN 2	
	AMOUNT	CALORIES	AMOUNT	CALORIES
Lean beef	2 oz	140	3 oz	210
Calf liver	2 oz	135	3 oz	197
Veal cutlet	2 oz	127	3 oz	191
Lamb chop, lean	2 oz	132	3 oz	198
Leg of lamb	2 oz	106	4 oz	212
Chicken	3 oz	115	5 oz	190
Game hen	3 oz	120	5 oz	200
Turkey	2 oz	146	3 oz	213
Salmon	3 oz	147	4 oz	196
Trout	4 oz	108	8 oz	216
Shad	2 oz	110	4 oz	220
Tuna	2 oz	107	4 oz	214
Swordfish	3 oz	144	4 oz	184
Cod	6 oz	120	10 oz	200
Halibut	4 oz	137	6 oz	204
Flounder	2 oz	112	4 oz	224

NOTE: I recommend having the main protein of the day and the main starch t different meals, so you will eat more vegetables, which are extremely important in my diet. Have 1 protein per day or smaller portions of 2 proteins.

NATURAL SWEETENERS CHART

	COLUMN 1	COLUMN 2
	CALORIES/ TABLESPOON	CALORIES/ TEASPOON
Maple syrup	64	21
Honey	80	27
Molasses	67	22
Carob powder	18	6
Apple concentrate	60	20
Cherry concentrate	56	19
Grape concentrate	72	24
Dates, dried, chopped	46	15
Figs, dried, chopped	42	14
Prunes	44	15
Raisins	44	15
Apricots, dried	39	13
Pears, dried	19	6

NOTE: Be very sparing in your use of these concentrated sweeteners.

NUTS AND SEEDS

You can purchase raw nut and seed butters at most health food stores or if you have a Champion Juicer, you can make them yourself. They make wonderful snack spreads, salad dressings (diluted) and blender drinks with milk, apple juice, pineapple juice, carrot juice or herbal teas.

Alternatively, you can grind up nuts and seeds finely in a blender to sprinkle on salads, cooked vegetables, whole grain cereals, soups and other dishes to add nutritional value. Nuts and seeds are high in calcium, phosphorus, iron and potassium and have a sprinkling of the B vitamins. There is no cholesterol in the oils found in nuts and seeds.

RAW NUTS AND SEEDS CHART: BUTTERS AND FINE GRINDS

	COLUMN 1	COLUMN 2
	CALORIES/TABLESPOON	CALORIES/TEASPOON
Almonds	90	30
Cashews	85	28
Pecans	103	34
Hazelnuts	98	33
Walnuts	98	33
Sesame seeds	22	7
Sunflower seeds	84	28
Pumpkin seeds (pepitas)	83	28

NOTE: Nut and seed butters can be added to broths and soups to increase their protein value. Finely-ground nuts and seeds can be sprinkled on cereals, salads, hot vegetables—almost any food, in fact. We get our finest oils from seeds and nuts for building the nerves, glands and brain.

SALAD CHART

	AMOUNT	CALORIES
Mixed vegetables (6-8)	2 cups	50
Coleslaw (with dressing)	1 cup	151
Carrot/raisin	1 cup	204
Cucumber/yogurt dressing	1 cup	90
Gelatin with fruit	6 oz	120
Gelatin with vegetables	6 oz	110
Waldorf salad	6 oz	170
Mixed fruit	6 oz	170

For mixed raw vegetable salad, I suggest a combination of at least six of the following: Romaine, red leaf lettuce, butter lettuce, celery, radishes, cucumber, tomato, parsley, green onions, green bell pepper, watercress, endive, broccoli bits and cauliflower bits. Grate raw carrot, beet, turnip and/or parsnip on top to make it a rainbow salad. If you use all the preceding, you'll have 18 vegetable in it!

DRESSINGS

	AMOUNT	CALORIES
Bleu cheese	1 tablespoon	76
French	1 tablespoon	62
Thousand Island	1 tablespoon	75
Vinegar and oil	1 tablespoon	83
Avocado	1/6 large	62
Roquefort	1 tablespoon	76
Italian	1 tablespoon	83
Mayonnaise	1 tablespoon	110
Lemon juice & oil	1 tablespoon	83
Herb, oil & vinegar*	1 tablespoon	83

*Herb, oil and vinegar dressing is made by using 3 parts cold pressed vegetable oil to 1 part wine vinegar, then adding any mixture of: garlic, parsley, fresh oregano, dill, sweet basil, thyme, grated lemon peel. Allow to age from 1-2 weeks.

SNACKS

You can arrange your snacks and snack times any way you wish, picking any combination from the list that adds up to the allowable snack calories per day. You can skip the morning snack and double up on the afternoon snack or vice versa, but I recommend against doing that with the evening snack. Evening snacks are more likely to turn to fat than any others. For that reason, I strongly recommend that you stick to such snacks as vegetables, broth, crackers and herb tea after dinner.

SNACK CHART

	CALORIES
FRUIT	
Small banana	80
Ripe orange, sections	80
Apple, half	60
Small, fresh fig	30
Large, dried fig	60
Half cantaloupe	60
Honeydew slice (10 oz)	70
Watermelon slice (10 oz)	75
Half large pear	70
Stewed prunes, 3	75
Raw pineapple cubes, 1 cup	75
Large peach	50
Cherries, 20	75
Half mango, 4 oz	70
Papaya, 7 oz	75
Guava, 4 oz	60
Strawberries, 1 cup	60
Medium plum	30
Dried dates, each	10
Ripe olives, each	13
DRINKS	
Herb tea	0
Broth, 1 cup	30
w/1 T lecithin granules	80
Coffee substitute	0
Carrot juice, 8 oz	50

NOTE: I am not encouraging snacks, but allowing them for those who have to have something extra. If you don't feel like a snack, don't have one.

(continued next page)

SNACKS (Cont'd)

	CALORIES
VEGETABLES	
Medium carrot	30
Medium tomato, sliced	35
Large celery stalk	5
Broccoli, 3 oz	30
Cucumber slices, each	1
Radishes, each	2
Sprouts, 1 cup	16
NUTS (Raw)	
Almonds, each	7
Cashews, each	8.5
Pecans, each	5
Walnuts, each	8
Sunflower seeds, 2 tablespoons	70
CRACKERS	
Ry-Krisp, 2	60
Sesame, 6	60
Ak-Mak	60
Ak-Mak, 4 squares	60
CHEESE	
Cheddar, 1/2 slice (1/2 oz)	56
Cream, 1 tablespoon	53
Cottage, 1/2 cup	60
Swiss, 1/2 slice (1/2 oz)	52
NUT AND SEED BUTTERS	
Almond	52
Cashew	35
Pumpkin seed	34
Sesame	19
Sunflower	35
Walnut	41
YOGURT, 1/3 cup	53
AVOCADO, 1/6 large	62

NOTE: Combinations such as nut butter and cheese, nut butter or cream cheese and celery, crackers and nut butter or cheese make satisfying snacks. Simply cut down the amount of each to fit the calorie requirement as necessary for a particular snack time. Use lettuce or zucchini instead of bread, and put snack fillers on them for a treat.

SOUP CHART

	AMOUNT	CALORIES
Beef broth	1 cup	30
Vegetable broth	1 cup	5
Chicken broth	1 cup	22
Split pea	1 cup	148
Vegetable soup	1 cup	80
Onion soup	1 cup	90
Lentil soup	1 cup	130

NOTE: To make a nice protein broth, add nut butter or tofu to broth. You can also add egg yolk, as the Chinese do.

BEST REDUCING FOODS IN MAGIC THREES
Cal/100 gm (or 3-1/2 oz)

BEST 3 Cereal Grains
Brown rice	87
Rye	81
Millet	78

BEST 3 Fruits (raw)
Cantaloupe	25
Watermelon	27
Strawberries	37

BEST 3 Soups (cal per cup)
Vegetable broth	5
Chicken broth	22
Vegetable soup	80

BEST 3 Snacks
Ry-Krisp (2)	60
Chico-San rice crackers	70
Sesame seed butter (1 T)	82

BEST 3 Natural Sweeteners
Honey	
Carob powder	18
Raisins	44

BEST 3 Proteins (broiled)
Halibut	130
Salmon (baked)	182
Chicken, roasted	199

BEST 3 Vegetables (raw)
Celery	13
Radish	17
Leaf lettuce (sprouts, watercress)	17

BEST 3 Vegetables (cooked)
Zucchini (steamed)	14
Broccoli	26
Green beans (beets and carrots)	25

BEST 3 Drinks
Tsp chlorophyll in cup of hot water	0
Herbal teas	0
Carrot juice (8 oz)	50

BEST 3 Seasonings
Vegetable broth powder (instead of salt)
Cayenne pepper (instead of black pepper)
Sweet basil

VEGETABLE CHART
(Cooked except as noted)

	AMOUNT	CALORIES
Artichoke	1 small	50
Asparagus	8 stalks	32
Beans, fresh	1/2 cup	15
Beans, lima	1/2 cup	80
Beets	1/2 cup	30
Beets, raw	tablespoon	5
Beet greens	1/2 cup	9
Broccoli	1/2 cup	20
Broccoli, raw	1/2 cup	27
Brussels sprouts	20	20
Cabbage, steamed	1/2 cup	34
Cabbage, raw	1/2 cup	12
Carrots	1/2 cup	24
Carrots, raw	1/2 cup	62
Carrot, raw	1 medium	30
Cauliflower	1/2 cup	10
Cauliflower, raw	1/2 cup	15
Celery	1/2 cup	8
Celery, raw	1/2 cup	6
Chives	1 tablespoon	3
Cob corn	1/2 ear	70
Corn kernels	1/2 cup	85
Cucumber	10 slices	10
Garlic	1 clove	6
Eggplant	1/2 cup	17
Kale	1/2 cup	16
Leaf lettuce	2 leaves	8
Leaf lettuce, raw	1 cup	16
Okra	1/2 cup	11
Onions, green, raw	6 each	20
Onions, mature	1/2 cup	25
Parsley, raw	1/2 cup	13
Parsnips	1/2 cup	53
Peas, fresh or frozen	1/2 cup	35
Peas, split	1/2 cup	115
Pepper, green, raw	1 medium	10
Radishes, raw	6 each	6
Spinach, raw or cooked	1/2 cup	20
Squash:		
Summer	1/2 cup	15
Winter	1/2 cup	39
Zucchini	1/2 cup	12
Zucchini, raw	1/2 cup	17
Butternut	1/2 cup	25
Tomatoes	1/2 cup	25
Tomatoes, raw	1 med	35

NOTE: These amounts make small portions which are adequate if you *use enough variety*. Variety is necessary to provide the body with all the chemical elements it needs.

MY SPECIAL TWO-WEEK DIET

This reducing diet is for 2 weeks. You are to have no dried or stewed fruit; have only fresh fruits. No pies, cakes, cookies, breads, ice cream or pastries of any kind are allowed.

Allowed Seasonings: Use herbs or broth seasoning. No salt.

Breads: Chico-San rice cakes (unsalted), Ry-Krisp (unsalted), Finn Crisp (rye).

Vegetable Broth: Potato peeling broth, vegetable broth. Broth seasoning can be made into a vegetable drink.

Desserts: Gelatin made with apple, cherry or grape concentrates or pineapple juice (with no added sugar). You may have this three times a week only.

Dressings: Tomato juice and avocado. Apple cider vinegar with 1 teaspoon sesame seed oil or honey. Apple cider vinegar, avocado and broth seasoning.

Fats: Butter, one teaspoon daily.

Beverages: Herb teas, vegetable broth, potato peeling broth, vegetable juices (fresh only), cereal coffee substitute—no sugar or cream.

To Control Appetite: One tablespoon whey in a vegetable drink or broth, 15 minutes before each meal.

MEAL SUGGESTIONS

BREAKFAST

Fresh fruit
Protein
Health drink

LUNCH

Vegetable salad (5 or 6 vegetables);
avocado every other day
Health drink

DINNER

Small salad
Two cooked vegetables
Protein
Health drink

164

FOOD SELECTIONS

FRUIT: Must be fresh—no dried fruits allowed.

Berries	Peaches
Melons	Pears
Cherries	Apricots
Grapes	Plums
Apples	Pineapple
Banana (1 per day)	Orange or grapefruit (sections only)
Papaya	Nectarines

Vegetables for Lunch Salad:

Parsley	Shredded beets*
Alfalfa sprouts	Carrots
Celery	Zucchini
Tomatoes	Leaf lettuce (No head lettuce)
Radishes	Endive
Cucumber	Watercress
Avocado	

*Have raw shredded beet—the size of a golfball—every day in your salads.

Cooked Vegetables (Steamed):

Fresh corn only	Beets
Spinach	Okra
Mushrooms	Celery
Yellow squash	Tomatoes
Summer squash	Cabbage
Snow peas	String beans
Brussels sprouts	Cauliflower
Turnips	Broccoli
Parsnips	Asparagus
Carrots	Onions
Banana squash	

Proteins:

    Meat (3 times a week only), bake, broil or roast
    Lean meat, no fat, no pork, no sausage
    Chicken or turkey (no skin)
    Lamb
    White fish or salmon
    Tofu
    Sesame seed butter
    Cottage cheese
    Yogurt

Special Supplements with Each Meal:

    4 Alfalfa tablets (crack before swallowing)
    2 Digestaids
    1 KB-11 herb tablet or tea
    1 Dulse tablet (have seaweed or a form of it every day)

Always think variety.

SUGGESTED MENUS

DAY 1

Breakfast
Nectarine—Peach—Apricots
1 or 2 soft-boiled eggs
Cleaver tea

Lunch
Vegetable salad—5 or 6, with color variety
Cooked brown rice
Alfalfa tea

Dinner
Small salad
Steamed asparagus and cauliflower
Broiled salmon
Papaya tea

DAY 2

Breakfast
Pears
2-egg omelet
Uva ursi tea

Lunch
Vegetable salad
Cooked millet
Mint tea

Dinner
Small salad
Corn-on-the-cob
Sliced tomatoes
Cottage cheese
Oat straw tea
Gelatin dessert

DAY 3

Breakfast
Orange—sections only
1 tbs Sesame seed butter
on Ry-Krisp or Chico-San
Shavegrass tea

Lunch
Vegetable salad
Cooked rye
Papaya tea

Dinner
Small salad
Steamed snow peas w/mushrooms
Baked chicken breast—no skin
Alfalfa tea

DAY 4

Breakfast
Grapes
1 or 2 poached eggs
Alfalfa tea

Lunch
Vegetable salad
Cooked yellow cornmeal
Shave grass tea

Dinner
Small salad
Steamed summer squash
Steamed spinach w/tofu
Uva ursi tea
Gelatin dessert
Sesame seed butter
w/Ry-Krisp or Chico-San
Oat straw tea

DAY 5

Breakfast
Banana
Cottage cheese
Papaya tea

Lunch
Vegetable salad
Cooked brown rice
Cleaver tea

Dinner
Small salad
Steamed cabbage
Steamed carrots

DAY 6

Breakfast
Apple
1- or 2-egg omelet
Oat straw tea

Lunch
Vegetable salad
Cooked millet
Uva ursi tea

Dinner
Small salad
Steamed okra
Steamed beets
Broiled lamb chop
Papaya tea
Gelatin dessert

DAY 7

Breakfast
Grapefruit—sections only
Plain yogurt
Lemon grass tea

Lunch
Vegetable salad
Cooked rye
Alfalfa tea

Dinner
Small salad
Steamed green beans
Steamed summer squash
Cottage cheese
Mint tea

DAY 8

Breakfast
Cherries
Cottage cheese
Mint tea

Lunch
Vegetable salad
Cooked brown rice
Oat straw tea

Dinner
Small salad
Corn-on-the-cob
Steamed asparagus
Sesame seed butter
Shavegrass tea
Gelatin dessert

DAY 9

Breakfast
Peach
1 or 2 soft-boiled eggs
Cleaver tea

Lunch
Vegetable salad
Baked banana squash
Lemon grass tea

Dinner
Small salad
Steamed parsnips
Steamed broccoli
Baked sea bass
Alfalfa tea

DAY 10

Breakfast
Banana
1 or 2 poached eggs
Uva ursi tea

Lunch
Vegetable salad
Cooked rye
Cleaver tea

Dinner
Small salad
Steamed Brussels sprouts
Steamed carrots & celery
Cottage cheese
Oat straw tea

DAY 11

Breakfast
Strawberries
Yogurt
Cleaver tea

Lunch
Vegetable salad
Cooked millet
Mint tea

Dinner
Small salad
Steamed spinach & onions
Broiled lean steak
Papaya tea

DAY 12

Breakfast
Pears
Plain yogurt
Alfa-mint tea

Lunch
Vegetable salad
Cooked yellow cornmeal
KB-11 herb tea

Dinner
Small salad
Steamed parsnips
Steamed snow peas
Tofu
Cleaver tea
Gelatin dessert

DAY 13

Breakfast
Orange sections
Cottage cheese
Oat straw tea

Lunch
Vegetable salad
Cooked brown rice
Shavegrass tea

Dinner
Small salad
Steamed beets
Steamed cauliflower
Baked turkey—no skin
Mint tea

DAY 14

Breakfast

Apricots
1- or 2-egg omelet
Lemon grass tea

Lunch

Vegetable salad
Cooked millet
Alfalfa tea

Dinner

Small salad
Steamed green beans
Steamed parsnips
Sesame seed butter
Shavegrass tea
Gelatin dessert

11

How to Help Overweight Children

About 12 million children and teenagers in the U.S. are overweight, and unless they are helped, many will turn into overweight adults. The National Children and Youth Fitness study of 10,000 children from 5 to 12 years old found that the average youngster is fatter and less physically fit than youngsters were 20 years ago.

Overweight children have a 50% risk of becoming overweight adults. The risk goes higher if an overweight child has one or both overweight parents. Assisting these children in losing weight is sensible, because the physical, chemical and stress factors that make obesity dangerous to the health are getting an earlier start and may lead to earlier health problems. It is easier to stick to a normal weight if careful food habits are encouraged early in life.

The Western Psychiatric Institute of the University of Pittsburg has developed a program for children up to age 12 that emphasizes diet, exercise and parental training.

PARENTAL TRAINING

Parents should set a good example by watching their own weight, eating right and exercising. They can also encourage and praise the child who is keeping to his or her diet and exercise program and reward them with gifts (*not food*) and special events like camping out, a trip to the zoo, a movie, the circus and so forth. Praise, encouragement and rewards help build and establish good diet and exercise habits. Parents can teach children games that make exercise fun and interesting. Overweight children need more encouragement and stimulation to exercise because it is harder for them, but as they gain skill and confidence, they begin to enjoy sports and exercises more.

TEACHING A CHILD GOOD DIET

A balanced diet, such as my Health and Harmony Food Regimen, is the starting point of the child's reducing program. Toddlers are generally taken care of by counting up the usual calorie intake and reducing it by 200 calories per day. Younger children will need a 900 to 1200 calorie intake, and teenagers will need 1200 calories. This should be worked out with your doctor.

Foods are divided into three categories—low calorie, average and high calorie. Low calorie foods are those 20 calories per serving or less (all vegetables) and are called "green light" or "green" foods for **go**. "Yellow" foods are those for which **caution** is needed, mostly foods in the middle range of calories in each food group: grains, fruits and vegetables, dairy products and meat, poultry and fish. "Red" foods are **stop** foods, the high calorie, fat-fried, sugar-saturated and junk foods.

Parents are in charge, most of the time, of what their children eat and how much is allowable in portion sizes. Mothers, particularly, but fathers too can take part in teaching children the *green, yellow* and *red* foods. With children, as with adults, meals within two or three hours of bedtime should be avoided. We have to realize that teenagers can't be pressured. Let them be responsible for their diets and exercise while setting a good example yourself. Praise them when they do well, encourage them when they forget, but avoid criticism. They simply don't respond to it. Teaching children to choose good foods and healthy activities can begin at age 5, in most cases. From ages 8 to 12, most can be taught the "game" of keeping records of their own food intake and exercise activities, but parents should still play a strong leading role.

CHILDREN AND EXERCISE

Many people, children included, find it hard to lose weight by simply eating less. That's why exercise is so important.

Encourage and teach your children activities and exercises they enjoy, and don't persist in trying to get them to do things beyond their level of skill or ability. Start easy and work them up to harder activities Do exercises with them. Take walks, play catch, go swimming. They will do things with you they won't do by themselves. Take them to playgrounds and pay attention to them as they climb on the monkey bars, slide down the slides and use the various items of play equipment. An adult's attention is a strong motivating factor in what and how much children will do. As they gain in skill and self-confidence in sports like skating, soccer, softball and others, they will begin doing more on their own, increasing in motivation.

BUILD A BETTER ATTITUDE

We do not try to treat obesity, because obesity is only a symptom. Our goal is to build toward a healthy lifestyle, so the whole body will be taken care of. Avoid teaching your child to focus on overweight as a problem, and instead teach him or her to have the healthiest body possible. Have a positive attitude and encourage a positive attitude in your children. When we teach children the value of a healthy body and how to make a healthy body, the weight problem is automatically taken care of in time.

12

Diets of the Stars

Many popular magazines and tabloids print the diets that famous TV and movie stars use to lose weight, telling the reader, "You, too, can shed unwanted ugly fat and look stunning by following the diets of the stars." Are these diets any good? Let's take a look.

First, we have to realize that the reason so many diet articles are being published is because everyone is looking for an easy, attractive, fast weight-loss diet. Secondly, the average person tends to believe that the stars' diets taste better and work faster than the diets most doctors know about, so many people take the stars' diets very seriously—at least until they've tried 3 or 4 of them. We have to realize that stars are not nutrition or diet experts.

Another thing we need to realize is that many of the popular stars lead unusually harsh, grueling lives. They are exposed to fatigue more often than most people, their working schedules are irregular and stressful, and we find that fame and constant media attention take their toll on a person's life. Most TV and movie stars do not live normal lives. Fatigue, stress, public exposure and fast living all tend to create acid conditions in the body, and this is especially true of the stars. So, weight-loss diets that are helpful to the stars may not be as helpful to the average person.

WHAT MAKES A GOOD DIET?

Let's review what goes into a healthy weight-loss program that takes off weight and keeps it off, then compare the stars' program with these principles.

For weight loss, calories in foods must be less than calories used in daily activities. The problem in the lifestyle or diet that brought on the weight gain in the first place should be resolved, and a more balanced diet and lifestyle taken on. Eliminate from the diet or greatly reduce, wheat, milk, sugar and most refined foods. Use the ratio of 6 vegetables, 2 fruits, 1 starch and 1 protein each day, with 60% raw foods, a variety of kinds of foods, no fatty pork or meat, no cooking in oil or grease, but emphasizing a balanced diet, regular exercise and a healthy way of life. These are the things we should look for in a healthy weight-loss program.

LOOKING OVER THE STARS' DIETS

Gavin McLeod, Captain of TV's "Love Boat," reportedly lost 34 pounds on a modified vegetarian diet after being overweight for 10 years. I like the abundance of fresh fruits, vegetables and whole grains in this 1,000-calorie-per day diet (sufficient for the average person), and avoidance of caffeine, alcohol and refined carbohydrates. However, I feel that skipping meals to speed up weight loss doesn't work well in most cases, because the thyroid gland slows down and we gain the weight back. Emphasis on milk products as a substitute for meat, fish, chicken and eggs is not good for those who are already milk logged, as most Americans are. This diet also recommends too much fruit, when we should be having 6 vegetables and 2 fruits per day or a 3-to-1 ratio of vegetables to fruits. Exercise isn't mentioned.

Elizabeth Taylor, one of the most beautiful film stars of our time lost 25 pounds in 45 days at the Betty Ford Center in California, using a diet recommended by the American Dietetic Association and the American Diabetes Association. While on the program, she was supervised by health-care professionals. The best side of this program was the variety of fruits, vegetables and lean meats offered, with emphasis on vegetable snacks and avoidance of caffeine, alcohol and commercial soft drinks. Not so good is the imbalance of fruits over vegetables overall and the lack of salads at mealtimes. We also find a number of refined wheat products, an overbalance of proteins and use of concentrated fats, which I do not believe in. Most of the starches were refined. There was no mention of exercise.

Dolly Parton, the famous country singer and film star, lost 5 pounds on a 48-hour diet, after going through a serious illness. This star was reported to be working so hard that she was taking prescription drugs to keep going, and it appears very much that she overworked her body and voice long past the fatigue point. Her 48-hour diet was almost completely fruitarian—melons, grapes, grapefruit, apples, bananas, chopped dates, figs and dried apricots, with a few finely chopped nuts. Allowed drinks were mineral water, herbal teas and fruit juices. Half a hardboiled egg, a little yogurt and 2 ounces of cooked shrimp were added to the second day's menu. This is a perfectly good diet for cleansing the kidneys and eliminating drug residues from the diet, but it is not a good weight-loss diet because it is so imbalanced and extreme. Most of the fruit found in stores is picked green to allow for shipping time, which is one reason I do not emphasize fruits in my program. This diet should not be used except under a doctor's supervision.

Victoria Principal, one of the stars of the TV series, "Dallas," presented what I consider to be a very good, balanced "30-day diet" for losing from 5 to 30 pounds. I like her emphasis on moderation and the lifestyle tips she presents. My only criticisms are that her diet is a little heavy on the protein side, a little light on the vegetable side and offers packaged breakfast cereals instead of the cooked whole-grain cereals. Exercise is a regular part of her program for staying in shape.

California's former governor, **Jerry Brown**, lost 35 pounds on the Pritikin diet, a low-fat, high-fiber diet program emphasizing fresh fruit, vegetables, whole-grain cereals, a little chicken and fish. This is a very fine diet, but hard for the average person to follow. For example, butter, all nuts but chestnuts, avocados, egg yolks and **all** sweeteners are excluded. Of course, it has been said that this is one of the best programs to take care of cardiovascular problems. The Pritikin program strongly emphasizes exercise.

Sharon Gless, costar of the TV series, "Cagney and Lacey," lost 45 pounds on a diet she calls her "yes-and-no" diet plan. At the end of her program, which included vigorous physical exercise, the 5-foot, 6-inch star weighed 125 pounds. She uses a simple list of "yes" and "no" foods to lose weight. The "yes" food list emphasizes vegetables, fruits, lean beef, chicken, turkey, fish, crab and shrimp. Drinks include skim milk, herb tea, water and decaffeinated coffee. The "no" list was not given. For the most part, I feel this is a good diet idea, but I do not approve of the proteins being served at nearly every meal (as they are in her plan) or of the whole wheat bread being the only whole grain cereal in the diet.

Wheat is the most fattening of the cereal grains, and most Americans eat too much of it. The interesting thing about Sharon's plan is her confession, "The minute we wrap any show, I dive into a plate of pasta." This may happen a great deal with show business people and is probably one of the "hazards" of the profession. This is a lifestyle problem of finding some more constructive response to the stress of finishing a show than by rewarding oneself with food (or alcohol or drugs, in other cases).

Jill Whelan, the "Love Boat" star who plays the Captain's daughter, Vickie, went up to 149 pounds by snacking on candy, cookies, pizza and desserts while working on the show. As in the case of Sharon Gless, this indicates a lifestyle problem. After consulting professional nutritionists, Jill lost 26 pounds in 2 months on a strict diet and strenuous exercise regimen. The emphasis in this diet was fruit, protein and drinking 10 glasses of water a day. The protein was fish only. I believe Jill responded to the need to lose weight in a very disciplined way, but we find that her diet lacked cereal grains, vegetables and variety in proteins. No one should follow such a diet without a doctor's supervision. It is too one-sided and comes considerably under the 1000-calories per day, considered the minimum calories needed for women.

Charlene Tilton of the TV show, "Dallas," lost 15 pounds on a 3-week crash diet emphasizing protein, fruit and 8 glasses of water a day. She also walks or jogs 2 miles a day, works out on gym equipment and takes tap dancing lessons. She has only a salad or piece of fruit, sometimes with yogurt, for lunch. I would not recommend this diet because it lacks vegetables, whole grains, balance and variety. This not a diet that shoud be used without a doctor's supervision.

When *David Hasselhoff*, star of the TV series, "Knight Rider," got married and honeymooned in Hawaii his weight increased to 198 pounds. In 30-days, he lost 18 pounds and 3 inches from his waist by following a routine diet of fruit for breakfast, protein and vegetables for lunch, the same combination for dinner as lunch, 8 to 12 glasses of water every day and vigorous exercise. Protein choices were fish and poultry, and no food was allowed after 7 pm. I like the separation of fruit and vegetables on this diet, and the limitation of lunch protein to make sure plenty of vegetables were taken. I also approve of the forbidden foods list: no alcohol, sugar, salt, canned foods, frozen foods or red meat. However, the lunch and dinner salads consisted of a quarter head of lettuce, which I feel is nutritionally worthless. Leaf lettuces are much richer in vitamins, minerals and chlorophyll than head lettuce. We find this diet imbalanced because it lacks whole grain cereals and starches, but another good point is that it omits milk, wheat and sugar—the "big three" most overused foods in the average American diet. Once a week, Hasselhoff ate only watermelon and drank only watermelon juice—a very good cleansing diet—especially good for the kidneys. The diet was admittedly a "quick weight-loss plan," and readers were urged not to use it as a long-term diet plan. Lastly, Hasselhoff was supervised by a fitness consultant, which is necessary when using any one-sided or fast weight-loss plans.

WEIGHT CONTROL AND THE STARS

We find that many stars have the same problems the average person has in trying to control weight. Here are some little-known facts about some famous stars, along with my comments.

Michael Landon eats one large meal a day and works out with weights to stay in shape. *Comment:* The metabolism of some people allows them to do well on one meal a day, but most people need two or three.

Barbra Streisand has had weight problems since her teens and first began dieting in high school. After a brief fling with fad diets (which made her feel terrible), she settled on a balanced diet with lots of salads, while avoiding fattening foods. **Comment:** The faster we get away from fad diets and into a right way of living, the better off we'll be.

Sally Field says, "I went on trillions of diets, but all my problems with food stemmed from emotions." **Comments:** This is true for many overweight persons and compulsive eaters, and unless we confront the emotional problems, we cannot control the weight. Sometimes it is best to seek professional counsel about the problem.

Luther Vandross, pop and soul star, lost 86 pounds in 7 months after giving up red meat, starchy foods (like bread and macaroni), sugary foods and salt. Vandross dropped from 315 pounds to 225 pounds using chicken, fish, vegetables and fruit. "The best part about losing weight is buying new clothes," he said. **Comment:** This is a great show of willpower. Since I don't have the proportions of Luther's diet, I can't say whether it is nicely balanced or not. He wants to lose 26 more pounds and I believe he will.

Melissa Gilbert, star of "Little House on the Prairie," says she is always on a diet, even though she exercises regularly and takes ballet.

Comment: When we encounter this kind of situation, we have to look at our lifestyle and attitudes toward food to see the problem. We need to get away from diets and find a right way of living.

Mike Farrell, "M.A.S.H." star, follows a natural food regimen as much as his acting career allows, and exercises regularly. **Comment:** This is the best and simplest way to stay healthy and maintain your natural weight.

Farrah Fawcett avoids white sugar, controls her meat consumption carefully, and eats lots of fruits and salads. **Comment:** Self-control and food control are two sides of the same coin, and we all need them to live healthy lives.

Jane Fonda was bulimic for many years, a subject that is still very sensitive with her. She finally overcame the problem with a vigorous, regular exercise program. **Comment:** It is possible that Jane's exercise program is too severe for many people, but there are some people who need this kind of program very much to show them they are capable of replacing a bad habit with a good one.

Janine Turner, TV star, eats three small meals a day and has her starch and protein at different meals. She drinks a lot of water each day. *Comment:* Many people eat far too much food for the work they do, and I feel this food regimen is very good. Separating the starch and protein also encourages us to eat more vegetables, and drinking plenty of pure water helps keep the body clean.

Lynda Carter says, "I keep a careful eye on my weight and never let it vary more than 5 pounds." When she gets overweight, she stops eating and takes only vitamins. **Comment:** I feel a short fast, supervised by a doctor, can be beneficial to the health many times, but we should not have to use fasting as a weight control method because it can be hard on the thyroid gland. Lifestyle is the key to proper weight control.

Dennis Weaver is a strong supporter of living a healthy lifestyle and using natural foods. *Comment:* I feel Dennis has found a balanced way of life, and show that it is possible to follow the path of health and have a successful acting career at the same time.

DIET-DOWNFALLS OF THE STARS

Like many dieters, stars that come off their diets often think of snacking or overindulging in foods that boosted their weight in the first place. Of course, it isn't what we do once in a while that causes problems, it's what we do every day, but the best solution to the problem of wanting the wrong foods is learning to enjoy and want non-fattening foods that are good for us. I find that many of my patients who stay with my Health and Harmony Food Regimen for six months or so often lose their cravings for salty foods, sugary foods and fatty foods.

Orson Welles, considered one of Hollywood's greatest geniuses, died in 1985 at the age of 70 after reaching nearly 400 pounds some months earlier. Welles was a chronic overeater who could put away several pounds of a gourmet beef dish and sweet desserts at a sitting, despite knowing that he had diabetes and a heart condition. Food was the only pleasure he had left in life, he once told a friend. Although he had successfully lost weight on several occasions over the years using diets, he always gained it back and more. **Comment:** Sometimes it's not what we eat that's the real problem, but what's eating us. Orson Welles never seemed to really find a proper outlet for his gifts, and I feel he was starving inside for something else besides food. It is very important for each of us to find our right path in life.

Elizabeth Taylor, after slimming down beautifully with a diet from the Betty Ford Center in California, took "time out" for a dinner of biscuits, fried chicken, gravy and mashed potatoes, with "mud pie" for dessert. This, of course, is a very fattening meal.

Bob Hope, who is 82 at the time of this writing, admits his weakness is lemon pie (which appens to be my favorite), but with the energy, vigor and wit he shows, I doubt that he strays much from a basically healthy food pattern.

Farrah Fawcett's favorite is bananas with ice cream, which is not bad as an occasional treat, if natural ice cream is used.

Vincent Price, star of so many horror films of past years, loves bread. "I can live on bread alone," he is quoted as saying. As I have repeatedly said in this book, Americans eat far too much wheat, and bread is used too much in the average diet. We should have the other whole grains like rice, corn and millet more often.

Charlene Tilton of "Dallas," whose reducing diet has already been discussed, loves banana splits with lots of syrup and whipped cream. If a person could eat a small banana split once in a while, it wouldn't be so bad, but the tendency is to eat large ones to the point of discomfort.

Lynda Carter of "Wonder Woman" loves beer, but limits the amount to preserve the slender shapeliness essential to her career.

Valerie Bertinelli of the TV show "One Day At A Time" has the most trouble with lasagna, one of her favorite foods.

Sharon Gless's diet, as previously discussed, helped her lose 45 pounds, but when she relaxes from a hard work session, she likes to unwind with pasta. The nicest thing she could do for herself would be to find a non-wheat food to unwind with.

Erik Estrada of CHIPs loves chocolate—chocolate cake, chocolate pies and chocolate chip ice cream. The problem with chocolate is its harmful effect on the bowel flora. Carob would be a much better treat for him.

Again, I want to emphasize that I don't seriously object to departing from a balanced, healthy food program once in a while. But I would like to get the idea across that some very lovely treats and desserts can be made from **NATURAL, WHOLE, PURE FOODS**, like carob, honey, dried fruit, fresh fruit, nuts and milk.

George Hamilton, for example, snacks on fruit. *Stepfanie Kramer* of "Hunter" eats cheese and raw nuts at break time. *Bob Hope,* despite his liking for lemon pie, more generally snacks on a bowl of stewed fruit such as peaches, pears or plums. *Don Stroud* of the TV series "Mike Hammer" eats a cup of kelp each day, which is high in iodine and trace elements from the sea.

IT ISN'T A MATTER OF *WHO* IS RIGHT BUT *WHAT* IS RIGHT

There are gourmet diets that emphasize natural foods. Some people have to stuff mushrooms, braise the endive or even broil grapefruit. There is nothing wrong with adding a touch of elegance to a natural diet and have more enjoyment as your body molds to better foods.

Jane Fonda has described how she alternately binged and purged herself with foods for 23 years before turning to a healthy way of life. Now 47 years old, in wonderful physical condition, Ms. Fonda is a physical fitness expert, as well as an actress. We find that fad diets, whether from Hollywood or anywhere else, may encourage eating disorders. We have to come back to the normal and the natural.

There are good "star" diets. In regard to *Jane Badler*, star of the TV series "V," there are many good things about the Way of Life diet designed by her mother that we would just like to mention. Using yogurt, fresh fruits, vegetables and other quality foods in proper proportions is wonderful. Bamboo sprouts have vitamins, silicon and fiber. People should use more sprouts of all kinds because they are low in calories and provide fiber to keep the bowel healthy. There's a lot of nourishment in them. Ms. Badler separates starches and proteins, and I think that is a good suggestion. Her diet is excellent.

People respond to diets differently. Some people are built like racehorses. You can feed them all day long and they never put on a pound! The ribs of some of those horses are showing all the time. Other horses eat a little grain and get so fat they are too sluggish to ride. Never follow anyone who says, "I can eat anything and it doesn't bother me." That's how people get into trouble. Let's find out **what** is right and not **who** is right.

I have had a lot of experience with overweight people who have taken off a pound a week by dieting, and in one year, a person can lose about 50 pounds. The wonderful thing about it is that they restored a good body, and they were able to keep their weight down by just eating the right foods.

The Weight Watchers' new "fun" diet has a lot of good points in it, showing what foods we can have over a period of one day. Of course, they encourage using skim milk, while I would suggest yogurt. *I believe whole, natural, pure foods are best for us,* and I would not recommend pickles to please anyone. I would rather make sure we stick to the natural as much as possible.

Happiness comes to us when we feel well, but so many people are living a moody life because they aren't using foods that feed the vital organs, glands and tissues properly. They don't have a good balance of nutrients in the bloodstream. They are one-sided persons; they think one sided; they act one-sided. Some become double personalities like Dr. Jeckyll and Mr. Hyde. We find these conditions are not necessary when we are living right.

Some people diet and exercise so they can have a sexier body. This isn't going to hurt anybody, but if you are living right, you don't have to worry about your body. A naturally healthy body is a naturally sexy body, the best body you can have. Besides, each body is unique. No two people's minds are the same. No two people's glands are the same. For these reasons, we have to eat according to our individual needs. If somebody could find a diet that would increase the sex appeal dramatically, everyone would go on that type of diet. But, in my program, we are going for balance, and the balance has to be measured by nutritional values.

All in all, when you look at so many of the stars' diets, it is well that we consider the natural and unnatural aspects. We consider the excess or deficiency of calories. We consider whether the food combinations are good or bad. We consider when a person eats during the day, how many meals he has, how many snacks he nibbles between meals. We consider what is prompting the excess eating, what is causing the weight gain. These are all part of my patients' problems, and I could add more. I realize that problems come from bad eating. So what are we going to do first? Are we going to take care of it mentally or physically? We have to take care of it both ways. It's a mental and physical problem. Most of the diets of the stars are directed toward restoring temporary physical beauty not health nor long-term well-being. This is something to think about.

13

Concluding Thoughts

Let's not fool ourselves. It is not the diet program that loses weight; it is the person who uses the diet program. Your body is designed to operate in accordance with certain natural laws, and only when you live in obedience to those laws, respecting the basic integrity and needs of your body, will you look and feel your very best.

My reducing diet plan avoids the extreme ways. If you follow it diligently and make the changes I have suggested in your lifestyle, you should be able to control your weight without difficulty. Overcoming weight problems requires paying attention to the whole person—body, mind and spirit—not just the symptom of unsightly bulges in the wrong places. Fat is a symptom that something is wrong in the body or lifestyle, and diets that treat only the symptom will fail. My plan works because we are taking care of the causes of weight and health problems, not the side effects of those causes.

Remember, if you are over 40 years of age or if you have chronic disease, it is an absolute must that you see a doctor and discuss your plans to lose weight with him. Reducing diets can be very dangerous when certain ailments are present such as diabetes, hypoglycemia and heart disease. Don't take chances. See a doctor and get counseling before beginning your reducing diet.

Overeating is the most obvious cause of obesity, and when overeating is simply due to carelessness in eating habits, the problem can be most easily taken care of. Keep a notebook or diary of what you eat and the times you eat for one month; this will help you adapt to more controlled eating habits. If the overeating is due to unhappiness or boredom, you will need to take a different approach. You may have to resolve a longstanding marriage problem, let go of an old grudge, change jobs or find more fulfilling activities to break the overeating habit. If the weight problem is due to organic causes, your doctor can help you find the best way to take care of it.

I often recommend several laboratory tests which can be helpful, and you should consult with your doctor on whether to use them. A thyroid test will show whether your thyroid gland may be contributing to your weight problem. The S.M.A. Panel, complete blood count and urinalysis provide a good deal of information about your state of health. If there are imbalances or deficiencies, it is best to know. My *Health and Harmony Food Regimen* will help overcome most imbalances, mineral deficiencies and other lifestyle-related problems.

Whether the overeating came first or some other problem caused it, the consequent obesity has caused certain imbalances in body chemistry and functions. Reducing may bring about periods of discomfort as organs and tissues throw off old toxins in the processes of burning up fat and replacing old tissue with new tissue, but these periods do not usually last long if they are natural healing crises or elimination processes. If the discomfort becomes severe or persists, check with your doctor.

Don't allow yourself to become bothered by teasing from relatives. Perhaps you have dieted before and gained it all back. Don't let the family needle you into thinking that's what will happen again. My reducing plan will not result in rebound weight gain if you follow instructions and change to a healthier lifestyle.

Avoid the temptation to lose weight as fast as possible. I realize how satisfying it is to see the bathroom scale show a loss of a pound a day or more, but burning off fat that fast generates ketone bodies, fat breakdown products which can damage the liver. And, high protein reducing diets generally result in unassimilated protein breakdown products which can damage the kidneys, whether you are losing weight rapidly or slowly.

Remember, 95% of those who resort to fad diets gain it all back again, many times with a few extra pounds. Avoid any diet plan or pill when advertisements or labels use words like *super, powerful, miraculous, fabulous, sensational, thrilling, exciting, startling, breakthrough* and the like. These are aimed at people who don't know any better. You do now.

Snacking is probably the biggest problem for most overweight persons. One recent survey showed that 68% of all Americans snack between meals, and 58% had snacks before bedtime. Ironically, only 20%

said they were satisfied with their present weight. Of those surveyed, 41% were on diets, with 38% trying to lose more than 10 pounds. Can you see the problem here? It can be taken care of, and it must be taken care of. Those little between-meal and bedtime snacks act like time bombs, ticking away until the fat bomb explodes one day over the bathroom scale. Defuse it. Eliminate snacking or use nonfattening snacks.

SELECTED FAST FOODS (TO AVOID) WITH CALORIES

FOOD	CALORIES
Hot dog	291
Double hamburger	350
Quarter-pounder & cheese	521
French fries	220
Onion rings	341
Apple turnover	290
Chocolate cake	250
Jelly donut	275
Fish, chips & coleslaw (large)	1100
Half of 15-in. pizza	1200
Fried chicken (3 pieces)	660
Chocolate shake	365
Banana split	580
Hot fudge sundae	580
Small fruit sundae	190
Sugared donut	255

NOTE: Most of these foods are loaded with chemical additives, are fried in hot oil or grease, are served with bread or are loaded with sugar. It is very hard to select a healthy, balanced meal at a fast food restaurant.

For those who have tried everything and failed to lose weight or keep it off even under a doctor's supervision, surgery may be considered if the danger to health from obesity is great. Gastric partition, which staples the stomach to leave a smaller pouch for food, may result in a 30% weight loss. Small meals must be eaten thereafter. Bypass operations join the stomach to the small intestine so that half the length of the bowel is bypassed. 30% weight loss is common, but there can be serious long-term effects such as diarrhea, bloating, gas, sodium-potassium imbalance, joint pains, skin rash, liver damage and so on. Usually people over 50 years of age or over 330 pounds in weight are considered too risky for surgery.

BEST TIPS FOR SUCCESSFUL WEIGHT REDUCTION

1. Don't think you can lose weight faster by skipping breakfast or lunch. The body metabolism simply slows down and burns fewer calories. *Breakfast normalizes blood sugar levels for the day and is very important.*

2. If you eat out have a small salad at home first. Select something from the restaurant menu that is not fried, creamed, battered or sauteed. Don't order obviously fattening foods of any kind. Think about what you want to eat **before** going out.

3. *Serve your children healthy, low-fat meals.* Research has shown that young children on a high fat food routine may grow up into overweight adults even though they do not overeat.

4. *Deliberately visualize yourself as slim,* wearing smart new clothes, as often as you like. Read fashion magazines. Visit department stores and clothing stores to plan the outfits you'll want to buy when you reach your weight goal.

5. The best way to stop habitual use of a particular food or food group—such as peanuts, corn chips, potato chips, candy or ice cream—*is to stop cold. Don't try to taper off. Don't buy the stuff and don't have it in the house.*

6. Dr. Kenneth Cooper recommends having 25% of your caloric intake at breakfast, 50% at lunch and 25% at dinner. *Heavy meals eaten late in the day or early evening are more likely to turn to fat.*

7. *Search for low-calorie gourmet treats in delicatessens, supermarkets and health food stores.* Make eating properly more fun.

8. *It is often easier—even fun—to lose weight along with one or more other people.* Pick a friend who wants to lose weight (or several friends). Encourage one another, share good low-calorie food or meal ideas, compare notes on how you are doing.

9. *Don't take naps after meals,* or more of your food intake will turn to fat. Go for a walk if you can. Don't eat your evening meal or any heavy foods later than 3 hours before bedtime.

10. Whole grain brown rice and millet are the least fattening of the cereal grains and starches. *Use them more often than others.*

11. *Exercise at least one half hour every morning* to increase your rate of *calorie burning* for the whole day—faster weight loss. Work out to the perspiration point at least twice a week.

12. *Eat plenty of high-fiber foods*—whole cereal grains, fresh fruits and vegetables. Use a teaspoon or two of psyllium husks, rice bran or wheat bran with each low-fiber meal to increase bulk and hasten bowel transit time.

13. *Herbal diurectic teas such as KB-11 or Cleaver tea,* taken twice a day, help cleanse tissues and prevent excess water retention. To reduce water, you may take these in tablet form.

14. *Take 1 or 2 beet tablets with each meal* for a mild laxative effect and to stimulate the flow of bile from liver and gallbladder.

15. *Avoid all fried or greasy foods, sugar, alcohol, white flour products* and as many processed foods as possible.

16. *Think positively about your goals* and rehearse them often. Put a meaning to your efforts.

17. *Eliminate table salt,* or, if you must have it, use a little evaporated sea salt. Use vegetable substitutes or broth from the health food store.

18. *Take 1 or 2 Novia Scotia dulse tablets with each meal,* or sprinkle soups, salads and other foods liberally with dulse powder. Kelp can be used in the same way.

19. *Face and take care of any personal problems,* boredom or depression that encourages you to overeat. Psychosomatic problems may be helped by counseling.

20. *You may want to try 100 mg of Niacin per meal* and work up gradually (50 mg/wk) to 500 mg per meal to flush the surface blood capilaries at the extremities and carry away toxic materials and fatty breakdown products. *Always take after a meal.*

21. *Use plenty of raw foods*—60% of your daily food, at least.

22. Realize that it is all right to be hungry and skip a meal.

23. *Don't eat meals by the clock*—wait until you are hungry.

24. *A sauna or steam bath twice a week to the point of perspiration will help.* Don't drink plain water afterward, but use a tsp. of broth powder in the water so the postassium will prevent excess water absorption.

25. If you use your credit card to charge fattening meals, *get rid of the card.*

26. *Eat slowly*—put your knife and fork down between bites to give yourself time to feel full before you overeat. *Remember, it is okay to stop eating before you feel full.*

27. *Thiamine, a B-complex vitamin which helps convert food to energy,* may assist weight loss. Cod liver oil (2 capsules a day) and vitamin C will help support the immune system as you lose weight.

Remember, a permanent change to a more natural lifestyle is the key to permanent weight control without dieting once you have reached the weight that is natural to your height and body frame. Good nutrition, adequate exercise and rest, positive thinking, good friends and relationships, loving yourself, a fulfilling occupation and home life—all these contribute importantly to your well being and to stabilized weight.

14

Things to Consider

I found the following interesting health facts in the process of keeping up with the latest news in the health arts, and I believe you will agree they are well worth sharing.

WHICH IS MORE FATTENING—STARCHES OR PROTEINS?

Ounce for ounce, starches and proteins have the same number of calories, and neither is more fattening than the other. It isn't so much the number of calories, and neither is more fattening than the other. It isn't so much the number of calories in a food that determines whether it is fattening, but how fast the calorie-carrying nutrients are released into the bloodstream. When the bloodstream is overloaded too quickly, the excess is stored as glycogen which can easily be turned into fat.

DOUBLE TROUBLE

A man who has commited a mistake and does not correct it is commiting another mistake.
—Confucius

WATCH OUT FOR DEFICIENCY SYMPTOMS

When you diet, watch out for dry skin, dull hair, cracked lips, white spots in the fingernails and muscle aches or cramps. These are signs that you may be deficient in certain vitamins and minerals. If you are faithfully followig the "Dr. Jensen Plan," then see your doctor for advice on additional supplements needed.

CONTROL OF FUTURE OBESITY IN BABIES

During the last few months of pregnancy, fat cells are manufactured in the fetus. Scientists found that babies of mothers who gained more than 40 pounds during pregnancy tend to have more fat than babies of mothers who have controlled their weight during pregnancy. The first year of a child's life, cells triple in number, and overfeeding at this time may be a major factor in later obesity by creating a larger-than-normal number of fat cells. Adolescence is another time when rapid growth takes place, and too much fatty food can again multiply the number of fat cells. The main difference between obese and non-obese people is the total number of fat cells, and by controlling the diet of the pregnant mother, the infant during the first year, and the teenager, scientists feel future obesity may be prevented.

BELIEVE IT OR NOT

The average persoin has 30 billion fat cells in the body, and gaining weight at first makes them larger. As the size limit is reached on existing fat cells, new ones are created until the total may approach 100 billion!

AMERICA'S FAVORITE PASTIME

A poll taken by Louis Harris in 1979 showed that eating was America's favorite leisure time activity. Of those surveyed 54% said they eat often while relaxing and another 30% occasionally ate to kill time. Take a walk!

CALORIE CONTEST

An eating contest in 1981 was won by Dee Dee Spencer in a little over 5 hours with a grand total of 42,194 calories, which included a German chocolate cake, 15 Twinkies, 14 cups of tuna salad, 16 cups of macaroni and cheese, 60 Oreo cookies and much, much more.

WHERE DO WE EAT?

Researchers have found that people who eat in only one or two rooms of the house (kitchen and dining room) have an easier time controlling their weight and food intake than those who eat in the living room, bedroom, den and other rooms of the house in addition to kitchen and dining room. Any room you eat in can become a "trigger" for impulsive snacking.

FEELING FULL ON LESS

To feel full on less food, eat slowly, put your fork or spoon down between bites, savor each bite and chew food thoroughly before swallowing. Don't watch TV or read books or magazines while you eat.

HOW FAT IS STORED

Studies of obese and non-obese people showed that the average amount of fat within each fat cell is 35% more in obese people. On the average, obese people had 3 times more fat cells than non-obese people. Researchers now believe there is an upper limit to the size fat cells can reach. After that, cells begin to divide, increasing in number to create new storage repositories for the fat that continues to come into the body. There are 5 miles of arteries and veins in every 5 pounds of fat tissue.

A panhandler had heard that fat women were a soft touch. Spying one, he went into his act.

"Lady," he begged, "Please have mercy on me. I haven't eaten in four days."

"My word," she gasped, "I wish I had your willpower!"

SHARE WITH YOUR FAMILY

When you go on a weight-loss diet, talk to your family, mention the foods you can't eat, and ask for their support and encouragement in your weight-loss goal. Dr. Michael LeBow says that support and encouragement from your family, mate and children help significantly in meeting dieting goals.

WORLD RECORD WEIGHT LOSS—925 LBS

The largest weight loss on record is that of a 1,400 pound cab driver, John Brower Minnock of Seattle, WA. After 15 months on a strict diet at Seattle's University Hospital, Minnoch dropped to 475 pounds. His goal is 210 pounds.

DIETING—WITH AND WITHOUT EXERCISE

A study by Dr. Neil Solomon, formerly of Johns Hopkins University, compared 61 dieters who exercised with 69 dieters who did not. The exercising dieters lost 20% more inches on the abdomen, buttocks and thighs than those who did not exercise.

SUPER MICRO-CALORIE REDUCING DIET

MONDAY

Breakfast	Weak tea
Lunch	1 bouillon cube in 1/2 cup diluted water
Dinner	1 pigeon thigh, 3 oz prune juice (gargle only)

TUESDAY

Breakfast	Scraped crumbs of burned toast
Lunch	1 doughnut hole (without sugar)
Dinner	2 jellyfish skins; 1 glass dehydrated water

WEDNESDAY

Breakfast	Boiled out stains from tablecloth
Lunch	1/2 doz poppy seeds
Dinner	Bees' knees & mosquito knuckles in vinegar

THURSDAY

Breakfast	1 lobster antennae
Lunch	1 guppy fin
Dinner	1 jellyfish vertebra ala mode

FRIDAY

Breakfast	2 shredded eggshell skins
Lunch	1 navel orange bellybutton
Dinner	3 Irish potato eyes

SATURDAY

Breakfast	4 chopped banana seeds
Lunch	1 broiled butterfly liver
Dinner	1 fillet of soft shell crab claw

SUNDAY

Breakfast	Pickled hummingbird tongue
Lunch	Prime rib of tadpole
Dinner	Tossed paprika and cloverleaf salad

NOTE: All meals are to be eaten under a microscope to avoid extra portions. No substitutions.

BEST DRINKS
FOR REDUCING

No-calorie drinks with a pleasing flavor: include a teaspoon of liquid chlorophyll in water (hot or cold), herbal teas and coffee substitutes made from roasted cereal grains and other vegetable sources and a watercress tablet (which is high in potassium to help rid tissues of water) crumbled into a glass of water. Those who tend to hold water in the tissues should never drink plain water. Recommended low-calorie drinks are herbal teas mixed with fruit or vegetable juice, herbal teas with a little honey, fruit juices diluted with water, and water with a little natural fruit concentrate (black cherry, apple and grape). Vegetable juices are less in calories and still better than fruit.

JUNK FOODS CAN
RUIN YOUR DIET

You can gain 15 pounds, even on a 1000-calorie-per-day reducing diet, if you include junk food such as candy, potato chips and donuts, according to Dr. H. L. Newbold. Many junk foods are not assimilated as nutrients but are turned into fat and stored instead.

SUPPLEMENTS IN DIETING

The USDA finds that women on low-calorie diets are likely to be deficient in calcium, magnesium, iron and vitamin B-6. Their official position is that anyone taking less than 1600 calories a day will have difficulty getting recommended levels of many nutrients.

HOW TO AVOID
OVERSNACKING

When you feel the urge to snack but know you shouldn't have the extra calories, here's how to control the snack habit.

1. Do something else—any activity to take your mind and attention off eating.

2. Delay 15 minutes before getting the snack, to prove to yourself you are in charge.

3. Eat snacks you don't really care for—carrots, celery, cucumber slices—in small amounts, chewing slowly.

4. Always take your snack to the eating area—kitchen, dining room, etc.—and sit down to eat.

5. Don't waste time feeling guilty about a snack, but get busy working or doing something right away.

MOST QUOTABLE QUOTE

"The United States is the only country in the Western world where there's a declining death rate for cardiovascular deaths," said Dr. Clyde Turner of Brooklyn, New York. He points out reduction in smoking, alcohol consumption and obesity as benefits of the public's health awareness.*

COLLEGE GIRLS UNHAPPY WITH THEIR FIGURES

A 1980 survey of college women reported in Science News found that 91% were unhappy with the way they looked. About 70% considered themselves overweight, when only 39% actually were, based on height and bone structure.

OVERWEIGHT TEENAGERS

Overweight teenagers are more likely to do something about their weight problem if the parents avoid trying to control or criticize the teenager's food habits, according to Dr Alvin N. Eden of New York University Medical Center. The best thing for parents to do is keep junk foods and fattening foods out of the house.

BECOMING OR STAYING SLIM

The best exercise for slimming is vigorous walking and the best time for maximum results is 1/2 hour before breakfast. Walking anytime is good for slimming. Walk to work if you can or park several blocks from your job and walk the rest of the way. When you go shopping, park at the back of the parking lot and walk more.

ANTACID PREPARATIONS, DO THEY WORK?

According to experts, over-the-counter antacid preparations may absorb stomach acids, but more acid is immediately secreted, so they are useless.

Remember that reducing is not a noble venture if you are ruining your health. We must keep good health in our minds at all times. A one-sided reducing diet will eventually cheat you of vitamins and minerals, then sickness can occur.

ALCOHOLIC DRINKS AND DIETING

Alcohol is surprisingly high in calories, which is why most sensible diets say to avoid it while trying to lose weight. A Tom Collins has 1809 calories and a 12-oz can of beer, about 140.

TIME & TIME AGAIN

According to Dr. Barbara Edelstein, the average American woman spends 12 weeks a year dieting. We find out when we are living right, we can do away with diets and still keep our weight down.

CEREAL GRAINS—ONE OF OUR BEST FOODS

The best nutritional and dollar-saving value is unrefined cooked cereal grains. Avoid the "instant" or "quick" cooking packaged hot cereals because processing has robbed them of nutrients, although they still have more food value than the "cold" breakfast cereals, which cost at least 50% more than unrefined cereals.

KEEP BUSY—SLIM FASTER

One of the best ways to make weight loss a pleasure instead of a burden is to plan activities in advance that will keep you busy and make you feel you have accomplished something worthwhile. Don't limit your activities to housework—do some things that get you out of the house, things that don't involve sitting and watching. A visit to an art gallery with a friend may involve an hour or more of walking and pleasant conversation. Or you could visit the zoo or an arboretum, go window shopping someplace you haven't been before. You know what you like to do—think about it—then do it.

ARE MORE EXPENSIVE CUTS OF BEEF LESS FATTENING?

Expensive cuts of beef taste better and are more tender because they are "marbled" with fat, and are more fattening than less expensive cuts of beef.

SKIPPING MEALS CAN INCREASE YOUR WEIGHT

Unless you are upset, ill or simply not hungry, it is not a good idea to skip meals. Skipping a meal causes the thyroid to slow down and the body uses fewer calories. The next time you eat, more of your food will turn to fat. Skipping meals lowers your blood sugar and energy, making you more easily subject to fatigue, depression and discouragement. Research has shown that skipping meals can actually slow down weight loss or even increase the weight, rather than helping you lose weight faster.

BEST CHANCES OF WEIGHT-LOSS EFFECTIVENESS

You are most likely to lose weight successfully, according to Dr. Charlotte Young at the Medical Nutrition Department at Cornell University, if you are: 1. emotionally well adjusted; 2. in the early stages of obesity; 3. an overweight adult who was not obese as a child; 4. not someone who has dieted before and failed or regained the lost weight; and 5. assured of one or more good reasons for wanting to lose weight.

DID YOU KNOW...?

The average person eating 2,800 calories a day or more would live longer and have fewer diseases if he or she cut the calories by 1/3 and the fat intake by 1/2, according to Dr. Robert Good of the Sloan-Kettering Cancer Center.

EAT LESS & LIVE LONGER

Researchers at the University of Notre Dame have discovered that people have a better chance of living a long, healthy life when you cut your food intake by 30% when you reach age 50.

If you are obese, it may be more than a dietetic problem. It is well to check with your doctor to see if there is any malfunction in the body. A complete clinical checkup is well for you if you are ill or not, and especially if you are obese.

THINK PINK FOR THINNESS

Staring at a 3-1/2 inch square of a certain shade of pink for about 5 minutes has helped hundreds of overweight persons lose weight and keep it off, according to Dr. Maria Simonson of the Health, Weight and Stress Program at Johns Hopkins University. When dieters crave a snack, they pick up the pink square and look at it. This shade, called "Baker-Miller pink" after the researchers who first tested it, apparently sends signals to the brain that reduce hunger. It is best used in combination with a balanced diet plan.

THE SECRET OF PERMANENT WEIGHT LOSS

It is better to concentrate on building a healthy body than to focus on diet or weight loss. When the body is properly taken care of, the symptom of excess weight will leave.

Vegetarian protein foods can be just as fattening as animal proteins, unless the diet is carefully balanced and overeating is controlled.

LET THE BEST COME FORTH

Many people overeat due to hidden frustration because their gifts and talents are not being expressed. Is there an artist inside you trying to break free? A musician longing to make beautiful music? Dramatic talent waiting to be expressed? Compassion for suffering people not yet put into service? Let the best in you come forth. "Man does not live by bread alone."

DAILY HEALTH REGIMEN

1. Start the day by drinking 2 or 3 glasses of water, one of them with a teaspoon of liquid chlorophyll.
2. Exercise, building up to 1/2 hour. (Can be walking.)
3. Breakfast (with supplements).
4. 10 AM: Fruit, herbal tea, broth or juice.
5. Lunch (with supplements).
6. 3 PM: Brief exercise period—stretching, bending or a short walk. Fruit snack allowed. 10-minute rest, lying down.
7. Dinner (with supplements). Do not eat later than 2-to-3 hours before bedtime. (Take a short walk after eating if possible.)

IS PROTEIN NON-FATTENING?

Consumption of extra protein has no benefits in weight-loss dieting, says a Federal Trade Commission report. Protein ingested in amounts greater than the body needs are catabolized and stored as fat.

EXERCISE, THE BEST FRIEND OF THE WEIGHT LOSS DIET

Dr. J. T. Cooper has found that a brisk 20-minute walk daily will burn up a pound a month, even without changing food intake. Exercise increases the flow of adrenaline, which reduces hunger and increases blood flow through the thyroid gland, which raises the metabolic level.

AT-HOME EXERCISES

At home there are many exercises you can do in the process of maintaining the house—bend over to pick up things, dust and vacuum energetically, do your mixing and chopping of foods by hand instead of using electrical appliances. All of these things burn up calories.

SUGARLESS GUM

Sugarless gum has about the same number of calories as regular gum in most cases. Read the label.

SAD BUT TRUE

As we grow older, eating the same amount of food will cause us to gradually put on weight. This is because we are less active when we are older, and our metabolilism or energy expenditure, also drops. This means we are burning fewer calories but eating the same, which goes directly into weight gain.

As stated in **Recommended Dietary Allowances** of the National Academy of Sciences, "A 1000-calorie weight-reduction diet, in order to be nutritionally adequate, would have to supply most nutrients in at least double the allowance per thousand calories, an objective this is difficult to achieve without supplementation."

FOOD AND YOUR GLANDS

An experiment in which prisoners of normal weight were paid to overeat showed that endocrine functions changed in nearly all of them. Endocrine imbalance often favors obesity, because hormones such as insulin, epinephrine, norepinephrine and others determine how food is used in the body. The condition is reversible, and all prisoners used in the test preferred to be thinner, so they returned to their normal weight.

THE WRONG KIND OF ENERGY CONSERVATION

There are 80 million or so overweight American men, women and teenagers conserving 203 billion pounds of fat, enough energy to power 900,000 cars for a year or provide enough electricity for a major city for four years!

It is possible those who are overweight have to work a little harder to be fit—from a physical standpoint—than the average person.

WHEN TO EAT, WHEN NOT TO EAT

Until you are hungry for the plainest foods, do not eat. Skip a meal if you are upset, overexcited, chilled, overheated, fatigued or just not feeling well.

QUICK CHECK ON YOUR WEIGHT

Men—To get your proper weight, start with 106 pounds and add 6 more pounds for every inch over 5 feet.

Women—Start with 105 and add 5 pounds for every inch you are over 5 feet tall.

SUGAR-COATED CEREALS

Most sugar-coated cereals have more sugar than people would add at home, and are much more expensive than if you sprinkled the sugar on yourself. The extra sugar spoils the taste buds and makes other foods seem bland and unappealing, especially for children.

Seek a competent nutritionist or doctor who knows nutrition to check on your idea of a well-fed, well-balanced eating regime in reducing, building, putting on weight or any ill health condition. Nutrition enters as No. 1 in our lifestyle of building.

Having a little protein or low-calorie starch with vegetables or fruits will not cause you to be hungry before the next meal.

Missing meals may not always be for your good. Try a healthful snack.

Do not have cheap food lunches or snacks. Spend your money on your foods or you will spend it on a doctor.

The kind of desserts and snacks you have may be a weight buildup. Watch them.

Apples are a good fiber food—and a good reducing snack—high in potassium also.

Vegetaranism does not mean just eating vegetables. A balance of all foods is necessary.

Fish does double duty in a reducing diet—it is low in calories and, in most cases, keeps us from cholesterol buildup.

CALORIE PINCHER AND A MEAL

Anytime you can add raw vegetables to your salads like radishes, asparagus, spinach, jicama, squash, summer squash, zucchini, onions, scallions, watercress, tomatoes, endive, mushrooms, celery, red cabbage, cucumbers, sprouts, you will find these are all low calorie, non-fattening foods. Proteins added like sardines, low-fat cheese bits, cottage cheese, chicken, eggs, turkey, fish, can almost make a meal.

WEIGHT LOSS
AND INFERTILITY

Too much weight loss can cause cessation of menstruation and infertility, says Dr. M.G.R. Hill of the University of Bristol in England. A study of 170 infertile women revealed that 39 had stopped ovulating because they had lost too much weight below their ideal body weight.

HOW MUCH IS ENOUGH?

The average American ate over 1,400 pounds of food in 1980, according to the U.S. Department of Agriculture.

TO CURB AN
EXCESSIVE APPETITE

Taking a teaspoon of honeybee pollen half an hour before a meal effectively reduces appetite and aids in weight loss.

VEGETARIAN DIET

Dutch scientists at Leiden University found that a vegetarian diet low in cholesterol might slow or stop fatty deposit buildup in the arteries.

DIET DIARY

Studies have shown that keeping a food diary for a few months is one of the most effective aids in permanent weight control. Write down everything you eat, when, where, with whom and what your feelings were at the time.

BREAST FEEDING
VS.
BOTTLE FEEDING

Breast-fed babies are less likely to become obese adults than bottle-fed babies. A breast-fed baby stops when he is full but bottle-fed babies are trained by mothers to drink the whole bottle. This teaches the child to ignore hunger signals and eat everything before him/her.

SECRET OF PERMANENT
WEIGHT-LOSS SUCCESS

The longer you keep your weight down after a weight-loss program, the easier it is to stay slender. The body and mind adapt to the "new you," and you get used to healthier eating habits without having to think about it. Temptation is greatest at first, so keep your chin up.

202

TAKE A BEFORE-BREAKFAST WALK TO SPEED WEIGHT LOSS

Researchers at Texas Women's University studied 35 overweight women and found that the women who walked 30 minutes before breakfast lost 42% more than a control group that didn't exercise and another control group that walked for 30 minutes before dinner.

THE LEAST HELPFUL EXERCISE

The least helpful exercise, according to the experts, is patting yourself on the back.

DIETING WITH YOUR SPOUSE

If you and your mate are going on the same weight-loss diet, both of you should realize that men tend to lose weight faster than women. That's because the body chemistry and metabolism are somewhat different between men and women. So, keep encouraging one another, and avoid teasing or envy if one loses weight more easily.

CAVE MAN DIET

Cave men ate as much meat as the average American, but it was wild game—only 4% fat as compared with 25-30% fat in today's beef. Cave men (and women) had twice as much fiber, 1/6 of the sodium and 4 times the vitamin C as most of us get.

THREE CHEERS FOR EXERCISE

The first cheer we should give for exercise is because it burns up fat calories while we are exercising. Cheer number two is deserved because exercise increases the metabolilc rate for up to 15 hours, burning extra calories all the while! Cheer number three is because exercise helps correct the biochemical imbalance that encourage fat production in the first place!

HEALTH HAZARDS— POT BELLIES

Pot-bellied people face greater risks of heart attacks and strokes, according to Dr. Ulf Smith of the University of Goteburg in Sweden.

PLANNING MAKES GOALS EASIER

Planning your diet meal program a week in advance has four big advantages. One: It puts food goals in your mind in advance, giving you a positive attitude toward success in weight loss. Two: It makes meal preparations easier during the week. Three: You don't have to think about food or food decisions as much. Four: Studies have shown that planned shopping cuts down on the food budget. Don't buy foods when you are extremely hungry—you will have a tendency to buy rich, fattening and soul satisfying foods.

WEIGHT LOSS MAY NOT BE STEADY

Weight loss is seldom regular, so don't be concerned if you lose less weight one week than another. Stick to your goals and your diet plan—and you'll lose the pounds and inches in good time. Be patient. Losing more than 2 pounds a week can result in rebound weight gain later.

SHOPPING TIPS

It's wiser to shop after you've eaten, to avoid impulse buying and tempting high calorie foods. Another good idea is to always use a shopping list, which helps save money and pick the foods you really need.

EXERCISE IMPROVES CALCIUM ABSORPTION

A recent survey showed that the average American woman over 40 is deficient in her daily calcium intake by 12%. Since exercise increases calcium absorption, it is especially necessary to get 20 minutes per day of some kind of exercise while dieting, which could further cut back calcium intake.

EXERCISE—THE BEST FRIEND OF THE WEIGHT LOSS DIET

Dr. J. T. Cooper has found that a brisk 20-minute walk a day will burn up a pound a month, even without changing food intake. Exercise increases the flow of adrenaline, which reduces hunger, and increases blood flow through the thyroid gland, which raises the metabolic level.

HERE IS

YOUR

BEAUTY BOOK

BONUS!

(You have earned it!)

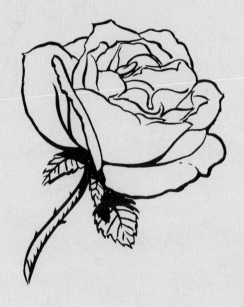

Dedicated to the "Beauty of the Rose"
that is part of the soul of everyone.

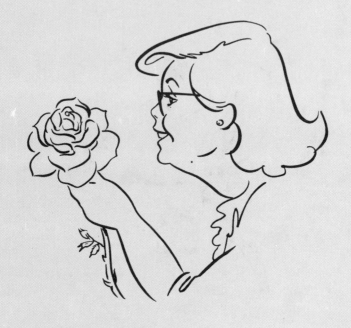

Hello, ladies,
I'm Anxious Ann
And I've simply
Got to find a plan

Introduction

To lose a few pounds is no problem, but to lose a few pounds *permanently* requires a plan. It is possible for you, through this complete *Beauty and Charm Plan* to accomplish your goal. Work with the plan and it will work for you.

Please understand that we are not trying to take the place of a doctor's professional advice. If excess fat is caused by pathological or diseased conditions, these cases respond much better under specific advice from your family physician. Consider our program to be that of teaching right-living habits. It is planned in such a way as to cause no discomfort of any kind; will not interfere with your daily routine and best of all—will help you build a healthy body.

Many have lost weight in a way which has proven detrimental to their health. Nature is health, and the healthy way is the *normal* way to reduce excess pounds while still retaining the rounded body contours that were meant for *YOU*.

Your greatest reducing aid is to follow a natural, simple way of eating. The simple, natural foods help to build a beautiful body by building a good bloodstream. To maintain a clean bloodstream, you *must* have good elimination.

The skin is a very important factor in your elimination. Two to four pounds of waste are eliminated through the skin daily, unless interfered with by excess fat.

It takes willpower to build lovely body contours. Strenghten this willpower each day and remember you cannot expect good results with the best guidance unless YOU have the *DESIRE* to accomplish your purpose. This desire comes through a change in your mental attitude. Greater beauty and more health can come to you when you stick to the right foods and control your daily habits of living. This is a goal worth working for.

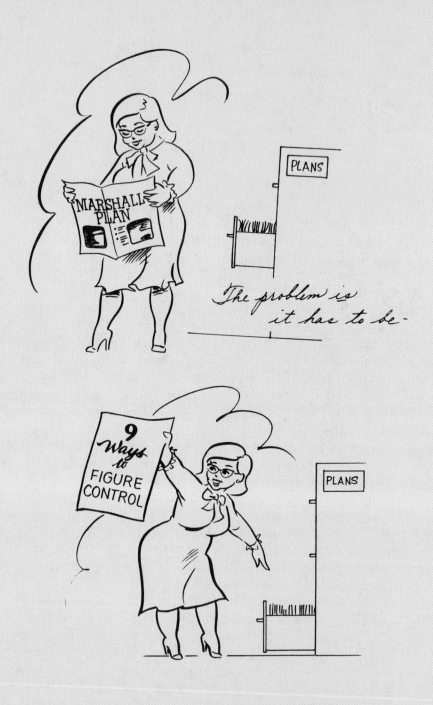

The problem is it has to be—

—just the right plan for both you and me

Through this simple 9-Way Living Lovelier Figure Control Program, you may lose excess weight and gain in poise and self-confidence, adding *LIFE TO YOUR DAYS AS WELL AS DAYS TO YOUR LIFE.*

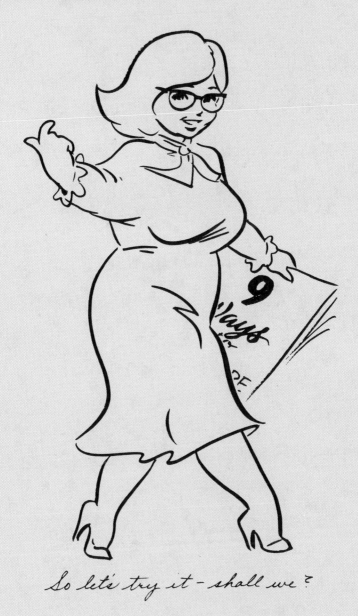

So let's try it – shall we?

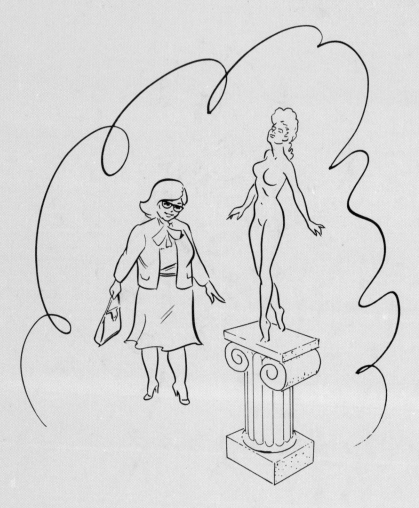

And I'm going to have
a figure as lovely as that!

BEAUTY BOOK CONTENTS

Chapter 1

Changing Your Mental Attitude

Every woman can do exactly what she wants to do. **YOU** can do what **YOU** want to do. You limit yourself by the way you think. When you find you really want to live lovelier you have begun to change your mental attitude but when you say you haven't time to improve your appearance, or that you can't do without certain foods, then you are hindering yourself. Anything *worth* having, requires effort to attain. You earn the right to a beautiful body through **EFFORT.**

Visualize yourself as you will look through your efforts— streamlined, poised and completely self-confident—and you have already made the first step toward your goal. Develop willpower in your body. Your willpower is in direct proportion to your tissue tone. Fleshy, flabby tissue lacks willpower to accomplish much. Be good to yourself. Take the opportunity **NOW** to work out this problem.

Every cell of your body is dependent upon the blood that circulates around it. The blood is the *river of life*. This blood gets its nutrients from the food you eat. What you put into your mouth today will be walking and talking tomorrow.

To keep the blood from becoming stagnant, daily physical exercise is necessary. The blood must flow freely into the cells to nourish them and drain them of toxic waste and accumulated acids. Take care of your elimination system, fill your lungs with fresh air and your body with sunshine.

FEAR DESTROYS BEAUTY

Avoid the negative emotins of fear, worry and regret. They have their detrimental effects on every cell of the body. **A**

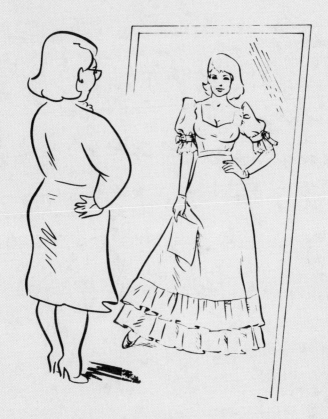

It may take a lot of persistence but I'm determined!

fearful body is not conducive to a beautiful body. Depression and melancholy often cause a sluggish liver and congested kidneys. Joy has the opposite effect. Joy gives the liver a "lift" and produces no acids for the kidneys to care for. Happiness is beauty in the body and exists both inside and outside. The happiness or unhappiness that grows within you is expressed on your face and reflects your well-being.

Think of your kitchen only as a "beauty room," and the meals you plan as "beauty treatments." Start thinking of yourself as the "new you" and re-educate your mind by changing your daily habits into permanent "health habits." Through your efforts, you will find the true *JOY OF LIVING*.

Oh oh! No more doughnuts for me if that's where they go

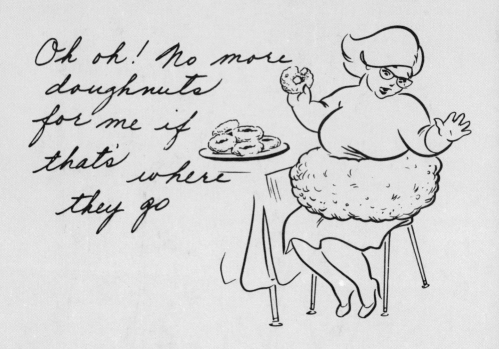

There are a few "don'ts" in the Nine Way plan but mostly there are wonderful things to do

BOARD OF RE-EDUCATION

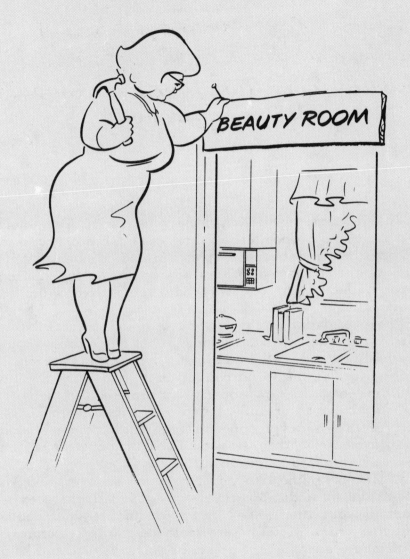

And this is where it all begins

Chapter 2

Control Your Glands or Your Glands Will Control You

The emotions, the diet and the nervous system all definitely affect the glands. When these factors are worked to excess in the body, the glands become depleted to such an extent that the body weight is affected. When the glands are functioning properly, the weight is right and beauty from within is experienced.

The thyroid gland is the "go-ahead" gland and is probably the most important of all the glands in controlling your weight. It burns up fat and is affected directly by toxins in the system. The best food in the world cannot be utilized if the thyroid gland is not working properly. Its unbalanced activity, whether overactive or underactive, may cause nervousness, heart trouble, lack of concentration, high or low blood pressure, menstrual disorders and a calcium deficiency in the body, in addition to weight disturbances.

A lack of iodine can develop either an overactive or underactive thyroid, and goiter may result. Include extra iodine in your diet when on a reducing regime. Foods particularly high in iodine are seafoods, garlic, watercress, onions and pineapple. Powdered dulse, sea lettuce and kelp are high in iodine and may be obtained in the health food stores.

The high starch and sugar diet of today produces excess fat which often causes kidney, heart and glandular disturbances (particularly the pancreas). A meal plan consisting of healthful, simple foods is a strong ally against these diseased conditions.

Thyroxin is the hormone manufactured by the thyroid gland which is so necessary to our metabolism, but hormones should be taken only on a doctor's prescription. The hormones from your glands will be secreted into your bloodstream naturally when you build up your health and develop a vitally-alive body of the proper weight.

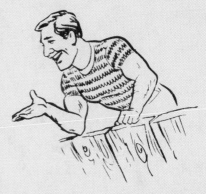

Hi, Chubby

It is important to learn how to free yourself from emotional strain, for this alone can develop a thyroid condition which is more difficult to overcome as your age increases. Your thinking is equally as important as the food you eat. Make every effort to free yourself of any anxiety, jealousy, resentment, hatred and fear as these emotions cause a lack of balance in the glandular system. Straighten out your thinking, and your beauty will shine from within.

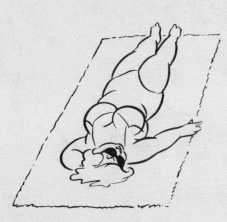

*Just wait—
I'll show him*

Think beautiful thoughts and you help to create a beautiful body. A good deal of beauty comes from *thinking* beauty. Poor body contours can be developed through bad thinking habits. Youthful, graceful thoughts help develop a youthful, graceful body.

To develop personality, balance your gland action by constructive thinking and eating habits. With a properly balanced glandular system,

you can promote unity and harmony both within your body
and in your environment.

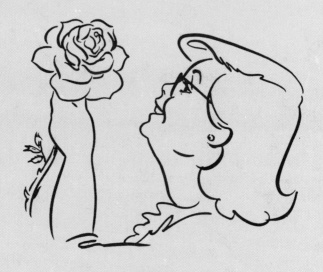

*Keep thinking beauty
and become beautiful*

Chapter 3

An "Organ Recital"

Interest and delight in the food you eat, is of primary importance in the digestion of your food. Consider not only a well-balanced meal but a zestful and appetizing one to help you in your figure transformation. Chew your food thoroughly to increase the flow of saliva. Prolonged chewing is necessary to help the digestive juices function properly. The stomach secretions are automatically increased as the food is swallowed. The food is then churned and segregated, and the process of breaking down the food for assimilation and elimination is well on its way.

There is a definite rhythmic relationship between digestion and elimination. Every part of the digestive system has a definite function toward making your food work for you, and, without the correct digestive processes, you cannot hope to obtain a good elimination. Faulty elimination means hoarding. You would not only be hoarding toxic wastes in your body, but hoarding extra pounds as well. Be interested in abdominal culture and intestinal management, and your weight will help normalize itself.

Infants usually move their bowels after every feeding. The normal bowel movement of an adult is the direct result of good care and training in childhood. This simple, mechanical process is correctly established and should be continued throughout a lifetime. The natural and automatic response of the large bowel to evacuate itself after each meal should take place, and will, if not inhibited by the distraction and rush of daily occupation or by sheer laziness. Fortunate are you who have been trained in childhood to heed this call and *promptly* respond to it! But for you who are not so fortunate, you can once again have normal bowel action through understanding the simple principles of elimination.

Let us list a few of the major causes of constipation:

1. Lack of exercise, particularly fresh-air exercise.
2. Worry, hurry and mental depression.
3. Insufficient green leafy vegetables and fruits.
4. Inadequate chewing of your food.
5. Not responding when the bowel impulse sounds its alarm.
6. Not sitting long enough for the bowel to empty itself thoroughly.
7. Taking too frequent laxatives and enemas.

To start a normal, daily bowel action in the new routine, you may use an occasional enema or a natural herb laxative. The herbs may be prepared as teas, if desired, senna leaves being one of the best. To prepare senna tea: Pour 1 pint boiling water over 1 tbsp senna leaves. Let stand 2 hours and then strain. Throw away the leaves and to the liquor, add an equal amount of prepared prune juice. Add 2 tbsp of honey after heating the combined liquids slightly. Drink a little of this juice after each meal or limit it only to the after-dinner meal, according to the looseness of the bowel.

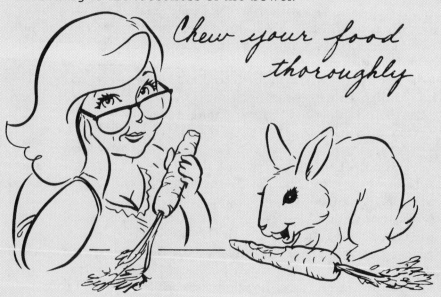

Chew your food thoroughly

The blood and every cell in your body are as clean as the eliminating organs. It is necessary that you keep the bowel in good working order so that the alimentary canal can be drained of toxic material properly.

You are a beautiful figure blessed when you possess a clear mind and a clean body as well. The mind is clear when the body has been cleansed of all toxic waste. With a clear mind and a clean body, you have the best chance for perfect health, a beautiful figure and a long life.

YOUR fountain of youth is merely a program of working close to nature by keeping your physical habits simple and wholesome. Depend on nature's way for your energy, vim and vigor, and weight-gaining habits will be banished forever.

"It is by a knowledge of diet that we take our fate out of the hands of chance."

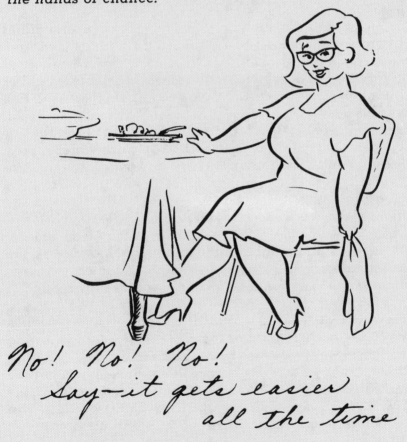

*No! No! No!
Say—it gets easier
all the time*

Chapter 4

Select Your Own Menu Plan

To make it easier for you to solve your own individual weight problem here are two food plans from which to make a selection. Each plan, or choice, has examples of balanced menus for three days, with the calories worked out for you. The total number of calories for each day in Choice I is 1000. Choice II is 1100.

Make your choice according to the amount of weight you wish to lose weekly, but be guided by your individual energy and occupation—whether a professional woman, a housewife or a woman who can give her entire time and energy to a reducing program.

Those of you who have more fat to lose or who want to lose it more quickly will follow Choice I. This is the "lean but not famished" plan and, although the quantity of food is less, the menus included in this plan are strength-and-energy-giving. In Choice II, the food intake is greater so your weight reduction will be slower.

Those of you who are following Choice I, may want a Choice II day occasionally or those of you who are following Choice II may want a Choice I day. Alternate the meal plan you have selected, if you wish, or mix them. Remember that the **VARIETY** of foods listed in these plans is essential. Limit the **QUANTITY** for speedier weight loss. The procedure you choose determines how much you lose. It's all up to you!

A lunch for loveliness and you are invited

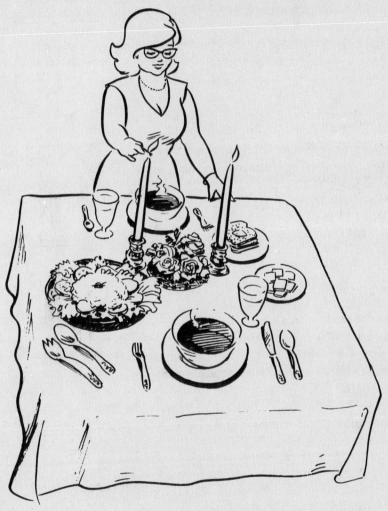

MENU PLAN
Choice I—1000 Calories

FIRST DAY

Breakfast	Calories	Total
Grapefruit (unsweetened)	50	
Apples (2)	120	
Skim milk (1 glass)	90	
Coffee substitute or herb tea	10	
		270

Lunch	Calories	Total
Two-egg omelet w/chopped chives (1 T)	165	
Coleslaw (1 C) w/lemon (1 t) and sour cream (1 T) dressing	80	
Melba toast (2)	90	
Butter (1/2 pat)	40	
Herb tea	0	
		375

Dinner	Calories	Total
Clear tomato soup (1 C)	165	
White fish (4 oz, broiled or baked) w/sliced onion and parsley	45	
Asparagus (8 stalks) and steamed Swiss chard (2/3 C)	50	
Butter (1/2 pat)	40	
Buttermilk (2/3 glass)	55	
		355

Calorie Daily Total: 1000

MENU PLAN
Choice I—1000 Calories

SECOND DAY

Breakfast	Calories	Total
Fresh fruit (choice of 2)	120	
Wholewheat toast (1 slice)	60	
Butter (1/2 pat)	40	
Skim milk (1 glass)	90	
Coffee substitute or herb tea	10	
		320

Lunch

	Calories	Total
Vegetable broth (1 C)	50	
Salad of sliced tomato, leaf lettuce, cottage cheese (4 oz dry style)	170	
Buttermilk (1 glass)	85	
		305

Dinner

	Calories	Total
Clear consomme (1 C)	30	
Lean meat (3-4 oz, roasted or broiled)	175	
Steamed greens (1/2 C) and cauliflower (1/2 small head)	80	
Butter (1/2 pat)	40	
Salad of watercress (1/2 bunch), lemon and oil dressing (1 t each)	50	
Herb tea	0	
		375

Calorie Daily Total: 1000

MENU PLAN
Choice I—1000 Calories

THIRD DAY

Breakfast	Calories	Total
Grapefruit juice (unsweetened, 1/2 glass)	42	
Revived dried fruit (sml serving)	100	
Wholegrain cereal (1 serving) w/milk	120	
Butter (1/2 pat)	40	
Skim milk (1/2 glass)	45	
Coffee substitute or herb tea	10	
		357

Lunch		
Vegetable broth (1 C)	50	
Pan-broiled liver (3-4 oz)	150	
Green leafy salad served w/lemon and oil dressing (1 t each)	130	
Buttermilk (1/2 glass)	43	
		373

Dinner		
Broiled, lean steak (3-4 oz)	175	
Steamed string beans (2/3 C) and carrots (1/2 C)	55	
1 peach or 3 apricots	40	
Herb tea	0	
		270

Calorie Daily Total: 1000

MENU PLAN
Choice II—1100 Calories

FIRST DAY

Breakfast	Calories	Total
Tomato juice (1 glass)	50	
Berries in season (1 C)	60	
Wholewheat toast (2 slices)	120	
Butter (1/2 pat)	40	
Coffee substitute or herb tea	10	
		280

Lunch

	Calories	Total
Cottage cheese (4 oz, dry style) w/chopped chives or green onions	120	
Tossed salad: lettuce (4 lvs), cucumber (1/4), celery and tops (2 stalks), chopped parsley (1/4 C), tomato, honey and lemon dressing (1 t each)	95	
Skim milk (1 glass)	90	
Grapes (med bunch)	85	
		390

Dinner

	Calories	Total
Consomme (1 C)	30	
Lean, broiled steak (6 oz)	200	
Steamed vegetables, 1 leafy (2, 1/2 C ea)	70	
Butter (1/2 pat)	40	
Skim milk (1 glass)	90	
		430

Calorie Daily Total: 1100

MENU PLAN
Choice II—1100 Calories

SECOND DAY

Breakfast	Calories	Total
Pineapple juice (unsweetened, 1 glass)	140	
1 egg, poached or boiled	80	
Fresh fruit or sml service revived dried fruit	100	
Skim milk (1/2 glass)	45	
Coffee substitute or herb tea	10	
		375

Lunch		
Vegetable plate: Spinach or Swiss chard, string beans, shredded beets, crookneck squash w/onion (1 C each), baked potato	195	
Butter (1 pat)	80	
Skim milk or buttermilk (1/2 gl)	45	
Cherries (20)	70	
		390

Dinner		
Bouillon (1 C)	30	
Broiled, ground round steak (6 oz) (mix in wheat germ)	210	
Shredded salad of: cabbage (1/2 C), carrot (1 med), apple (1/2), served with lemon and honey dressing (1/2 t each)	95	
		335

Calorie Daily Total: 1100

B-24

MENU PLAN
Choice II—1100 Calories

THIRD DAY

Breakfast	Calories	Total
Prune or apple juice (1 gl)	140	
Fruit plate of: sliced orange, berries (1/2 C), revived dried figs (3), melon balls (1/2 C), sprinkled with banana flakes (1 T)	230	
Coffee substitute or herb tea	10	
		380

Lunch		
Green pepper omelet (1 egg, 1/4 green pepper)	90	
Salad of: sliced tomato, Romaine lettuce (1/4 head)	60	
Whole grain toast (1 slice)	60	
Butter (1/2 pat)	40	
Skim milk or buttermilk (2/3 gl)	55	
		305

Dinner		
Vegetable broth (1 C)	50	
Broiled halibut steak (4 oz) w/lemon and parsley	200	
Steamed green peas (1/3 C) and Brussels sprouts (5)	60	
Butter (1/2 pat)	40	
Salad of: lettuce (4 lvs), celery (1 stalk), cucumber (1/4 med), green onion (1), lemon & oil dressing (1 t ea)	65	
		415

Calorie Daily Total: 1100

Make your own menus after the third day, using the same kind of food you have been eating in this diet, having a variety. Or you may use the same diet over again. Try going on this low calorie diet for nine days or longer, if desired.

THE BEST PLAN

The best plan is to start with Choice I under Menu Plan for six days and then when finished, take Choice II for three days. A healthy eating regime follows, which you should live on after you get off this diet., Repeat the low calorie diet once a month for the next two or three months, or two or three times a year, depending upon weight.

Remember, this is a diet for reducing and for elimination purposes; this is not a healthy way to live continually.

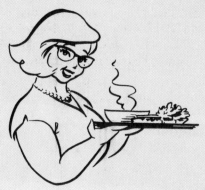

DR. JENSEN'S HEALTH AND HARMONY FOOD REGIMEN

Make a habit of applying the following general diet regimen to your everyday living. *THIS IS A HEALTHY WAY TO LIVE BECAUSE*, when followed, you do not have to think of vitamins, mineral elements or calories.

The best diet over a period of a day is 2 different fruits, at least 6 vegetables, 1 protein and 1 starch, with fruit or vegetable juices between meals. Eat at least 2 green leafy vegetables a day. Consider this regimen a dietetic law.

Before Breakfast. Upon arising, take any natural unsweetened fruit juice such as grapefruit, grape, pineapple or orange juice. This is to be taken one-half hour before breakfast.

Prune juice, fig juice, apple juice and black cherry juice are exceptionally good. Between fruit juice and breakfast follow this program:

Skin Brushing

Exercising, hiking, deep breathing or playing

Shower—start warm and cool off until your breath quickens. Never shower immediately upon arising.

Breakfast: Stewed fruit, one starch and health drink (See starches and health drinks listed under Lunch.) or **Two fruits, one protein and health drink.** Fruit of any kind, such as apricots, prunes, figs (stewed dried fruits), melon, grapes, peaches, pears, berries or baked apple, which may be sprinkled with some ground nuts or nut butter. If time of year suggests any other fruit, use it.

Suggestions: Sliced figs and cream; half cantaloupe with strawberries. Any TWO FRUITS with creamed cottage cheese and honey if you are a heavy worker and you feel as though fruit is not enough for you. Almond butter and cashew nut butter are quite nourishing and can be used on fruits. Eat an egg with fruit, and vary these from day to day.

10:30 am Health Drink

Lunch. Big raw salad, one starch, as listed, and **health drink**—with Rye Krisp, cornbread or bran muffins. Get salad suggestions from Dr. Jensen's book *Vital Foods for Total Health.*

Raw salad vegetables: tomatoes, lettuce, celery, cucumber, grated carrots, onions, cabbage, peppers, avocado, parsley, any raw salad vegetable.

Starch: Baked potato, baked banana (or at least dead ripe), cereals (whole grain), yellow cornmeal, millet, steamed brown rice or wild rice, steel-cut oatmeal, barley, buckwheat.

Drinks: Vegetable broths, coffee substitute, fruit or vegetable juices, oat straw tea, alfamint tea or any health drink.

3:00 pm. Fruit of any kind, such as dates, apples, figs, peaches, etc. Fruit juices or vegetable juices may also be taken.

Dinner. This meal should consist of a **small raw salad, two cooked vegetables, one protein and a broth or health drink**, if desired.

Cooked vegetables: peas, artichokes, carrots, beets, turnips, spinach, broccoli, beet tops, cauliflower, string beans, sprouts, cabbage, Swiss chard, eggplant, onions, zucchini, summer squash or any vegetable other than potatoes.

One Protein: ONCE A WEEK: FISH. Use white fish with fins and scales, such as sole, halibut, trout or sea trout. If complete vegetarian, use soybeans, lima beans, cottage cheese, etc. **THREE TIMES A WEEK: MEAT.** Use only poultry or lean meat. Never use pork or fats. If complete vegetarian, use soybeans, lima beans, cottage cheese, etc. **TWICE A WEEK: COTTAGE CHEESE,** and **ONCE A WEEK: OMELET.**

Drinks (broth or health beverage). If you have a protein at this meal, a health dessert is allowed but not recommended. *Do not eat protein and starch together. (Notice how they are separated.)*

You may exchange your noon meal for the evening meal— but follow same regimen. It takes exercise to handle raw food and we generally get more after our noon meal. That is why the big raw salad is advised at noon. Starches also need exercise, so if one eats sandwiches, it should be at noon. Never eat starch unless you have vegetables with it.

Fruit salads may be substituted for any of these meals. If you do not feel hungry or any too well, a fruit salad is the best food to eat.

Rules of Eating

1. If not entirely comfortable in mind and body from the previous mealtime, you should miss the next meal.

2. Do not eat unless you have a keen desire for the plainest food.

3. Do not eat beyond your needs.

4. Be sure to thoroughly masticate your food.

5. Miss meals if in pain—emotionally upset—not hungry, chilled, overheated and during acute illness.

Chapter 5

Your Body Alignment

Another important step in the attainment of figure charm—a step that goes hand in hand with the food you eat, is to learn how to be gracefully supple. The "new you" you are visualizing in your mirror, is a body not only glowing with health, eyes radiant with the inner sparkle of the right mental attitude, but a body graceful in posture, without tension, with beautiful curves and perfect poise.

Bodily movement, "figure-tively" speaking, is very necessary in your rebuilding program. Many of us become sedentary in our habits and that is what makes the pounds gather in the most inactive places. But, before you even consider the various ways of taking off this weight, look to your posture. How do *YOU* stand? What posture do *YOU* maintain all day? Are you a "slumper," a "stooper," a "twister" while seated, standing or walking? Are you a "duck-waddler?" Every organ in your body has better function when you maintain good posture; your lungs get sufficient fresh air and you can breathe freely. Every muscle in your body becomes stronger; they are not used to the fatigue limit, and you are able to relax when you rest. One of the principle ingredients of health is a strong and supple body in perfect alignment. Straighten up!

Indian women have developed a streamlined form of posture by carrying burdens on their heads. Push your head straight up as if you were carrying a book or package on the top of your head. This will automatically lift the chest and the stomach. You will walk with more ease and grace. You will look charming because you will *feel* charming.

B-29

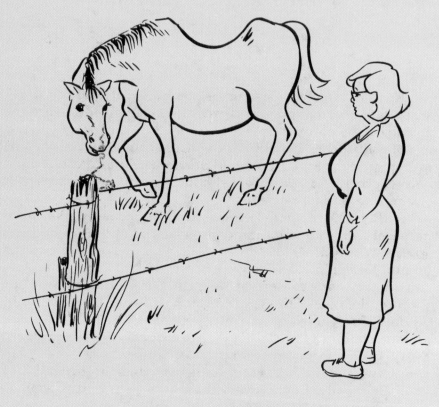

Poor thing!

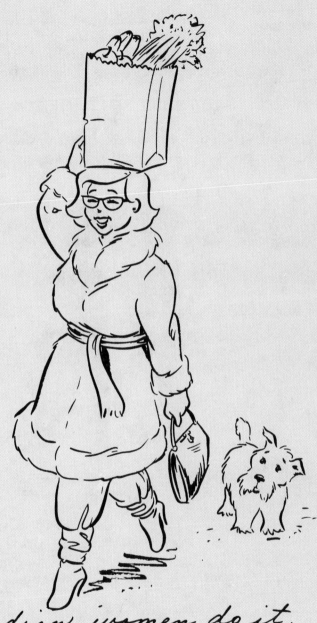

*Indian women do it.
And how well they
carry themselves*

B-31

To get your figure on a balanced plane, let an imaginary line go from the lobe of the ear, through the center of the shoulder, hip joint, knee and in front of the ankle bone. This line points out to you the proper goals to seek in body alignment.

EXERCISE AGAINST THE WALL FOR POSTURE

To help attain proper posture, stand against the wall, lower the hips and press the lower spine back against the wall, taking out the curve in the lower back. The stomach will fall into its

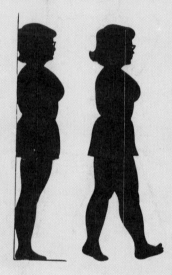

proper position of its own accord. Now walk away from the wall holding this position; exaggerate it for a while, until you can actually walk without that lower back curve.

Lining up the body in this way shows you how to keep the pubic bone tilted forward and upward while you are in a standing (or sitting) position. The buttocks tuck in automatically and the abnormal curvatures of the back straighten out.

Another exercise to help you is shown in the illustrations below.

Remember to carry the head high. Carry the chest high and stretch the body from the waistline to the base of the ribs. Keep your shoulders relaxed. You may feel an unnatural pull in the

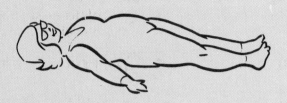

"Lie down - Insteps together"

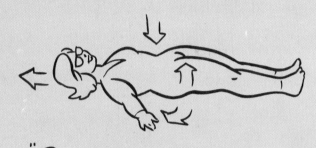

*"Pubic bone up - arms
out to side - stretch neck"*

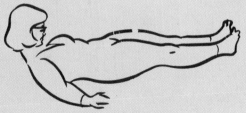

Oh, where is my tummy now?

thighs and knees. To counteract this pull, bend the knees slightly but hold the knees easily.

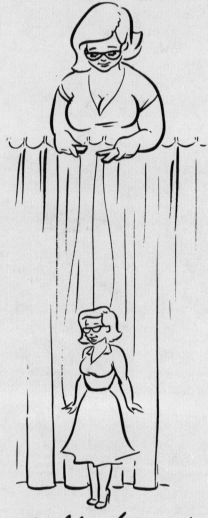

Feel the pull of an imaginary string to keep your body in perfect alignment

LEARN TO SIT CORRECTLY

Body alignment in a sitting position is just as important as in a standing position. *PUSH* the lower half of the spine against the chairback as you sit. Then line up the rest of the body. When sitting for long periods of time, tense and relax the hip and abdominal muscles vigorously. Feel the blood coursing through the lower extremities! This exercise not only awakens the blood but strengthens the flabby muscles that result in a "stenographer's spread."

Here is an exercise to help correct a poor posture: Lie flat on your back. Clasp your wrists under you as you arch your back. Return to the original position, relaxing completely. Repeat this exercise, with relaxation, 12 to 15 times.

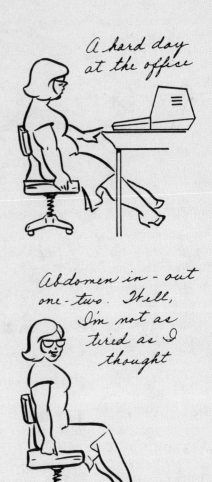

A hard day at the office

Abdomen in - out one - two. Well, I'm not as tired as I thought

Overweight shifts excessive strain onto the lower spine and the hip, knee and ankle joints, as well as causing excessive stress on supportive muscles and ligaments not designed to carry such strain. In time, these muscles and ligaments stretch and finally break down from fatigue. The body is not balanced in an erect position, and various bodily irritations result.

Old age is a state of "chronic fatigue." We are "old" when we are tired. We are tired because of improper posture and because we do not relax sufficiently. Relaxation is just as necessary as exercise to keep the body youthful. Tension,

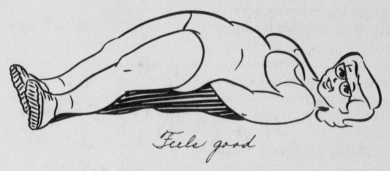

Feels good

alternating with relaxation in the body, is an excellent way to put tone and zip back into the muscles. Learn to tense and relax the muscles at will. Tensing and relaxing your muscles alternately not only "cleans house" within the muscle tissue but forces fresh blood and lymph to circulate.

BENEFITS OF THE SLANTING BOARD

One of the best methods of relaxation is lying flat in a slanting position, the feet higher than the head. You may wish to go through your body alignment program in this position. Accustom yourself to slanting board exercise and use your board just as regularly as you use your toothbrush. See Appendix on how to make your own slanting board. Exercises on this board both before and after periods of relaxation help to stimulate the blood circulation and reduce body weight.

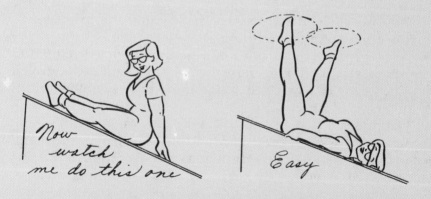

Now watch me do this one

Easy

One of the reasons why your abdomen may appear large and flabby is possibly because of a condition of prolapsus. This prolapsed position prevents the intestines from doing the natural work they are intended to do. This condition causes pressure on the kidneys, bladder and other pelvic organs, producing abnormalities of the female cycle that so many women experience. Before going to bed, lie on a slanting board to pull the organs back into position again. Do this consistently, to correct this condition, as well as to relax and align the body. Remember, too, that correct body alignment will help eliminate a bulgy abdomen.

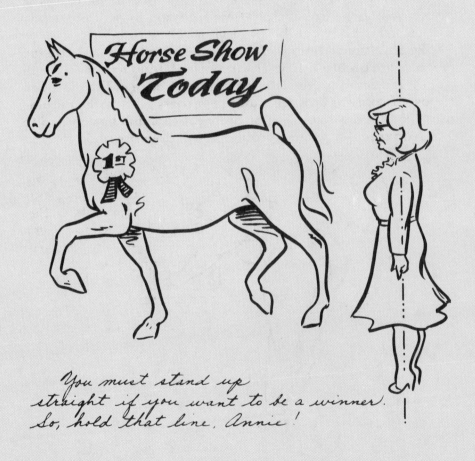

You must stand up straight if you want to be a winner. So, hold that line, Annie!

Chapter 6

Your Suppleness of Movement

Figure charm is expressed through your physical body. You may choose to have charm expressed in beautiful body curves. Your body can be what you want it to be.

Be ambitious about your figure, but don't try to take off too much in too great a hurry. The important thing to remember in weight reducing is *consistency* in the practice of the plan you choose. Twenty or thirty minutes spent every day in the regular practice of a few exercises or body movements best suited to *YOUR* particular weight problems will do more good for you

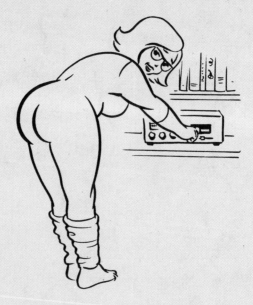

Now let's do these to music

than a greater time spent in scattered movements. Exercise that is not tiring but exhilarating is the activity to choose. Stimulate your sense of rhythm by doing these movements to music.

It is necessary that you engage in bodily activity to eliminate toxic wastes through the lungs and skin. Aerobic breathing and light perspiration, aided by good posture, helps eliminate toxins and acid wastes. A continuous supply of oxygen in the blood is important in breaking down fat, as oxygen helps burn up calories. Exercise develops tone in the tissues, makes the muscles more compact, and helps the body curves to become sleekly smooth!

The abdominal and back muscles are the most important ones to keep in condition. The vital organs are surrounded by

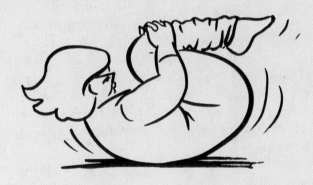

Rock a bye, Annie
It won't be too long
You'll have a fine figure
When the tummy muscles
get strong.

these muscles and it becomes almost physically impossible to have a prolapsed condition or for fat to accumulate, if these muscles have controlled strength.

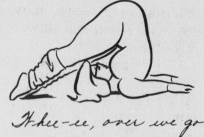

Whee-ee, over we go

A good exercise to stretch the spine and muscles of the abdomen is to (a) lie on your back on the floor, (b) grip the knees with the hands and rock backward and forward on the spine. The spine acts as a pivot. (c) After you have gained sufficient limberness, try touching your toes to the floor over your head.

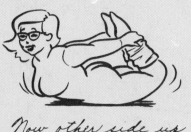

Now other side up

As an alternative exercise, the abdomen may be used as a pivot by rocking back and forth in a seesaw motion on your stomach while gripping your ankles, massaging the internal organs and strengthening the abdominal and back muscles.

Swimming is one of the best all-around activities as the body is in a prone position while exercising—an aid in reversing prolapsus. The bust is developed, and all the body muscles are brought into play.

If you are a "duck-waddler," one who walks with toes pointed out, *walk the line.* Follow a line in the sidewalk to help you learn to walk well or follow an imaginary line. This attention to your walking will help prevent your hips from wobbling and will smooth out your step.

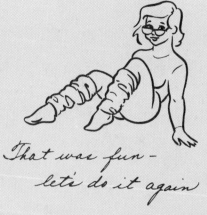

That was fun — let's do it again

Walk a little "pigeon-toed" to help correct the "toeing-out" manner of walking you may be using, which, in some cases, may cause an abnormal lower back curvature.

Try to avoid cramping your feet in shoes all day long and exercise daily without your shoes. Keep your feet limber by walking barefooted on your toes and work the muscles and arches of your feet as you walk. Walking barefoot on a sandy beach is one of the best ways to exercise and strengthen the feet and leg muscles. Dancing and massage are both excellent to help put spring in your step.

Your feet tell their troubles in your facial expressions. Keep your footprints off your face and remember, as you reduce, that your feet will appreciate the lighter load they carry. *(See Appendix for foot exercises.)*

Let us mention here, before talking about spot reducing, that the motions of the hands are a barometer of youth or old age. Jerky or aimless hand movements detract from an otherwise graceful body and add years to your appearance. Become conscious of your hand movements at all times and learn how to use them gracefully.

Hi

This does look better, doesn't it?

If the body is excessively large in any one spot, and the reducing diet and exercises you have chosen do not seem to reduce these spots, it may be necessary to include *spot reducing* in your program.

B-41

TO REDUCE THE NECK

1. Lie flat on the bed, floor or on your slanting board. Lift your head up until your chin touches your chest. Relax. Repeat six to ten times or until fatigued. This exercise helps to remove a double chin as well as reduce the neck.

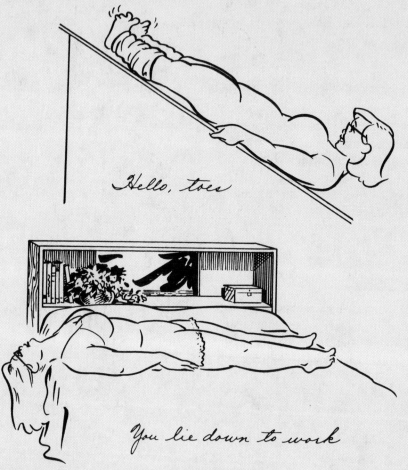

Hello, toes

You lie down to work

2. Lie flat on your back across the bed with your head hanging over the edge. Slowly lift your head until your chin touches your chest. Rotate your head slowly to the left, then up to the chest again. Then rotate your head slowly to the right and back to the chest again. Pause between movements to prevent overfatigue. Relax completely before repeating the entire

exercise. Reverse this procedure by lying face down on the bed, with the head hanging over the edge.

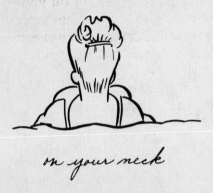

on your neck

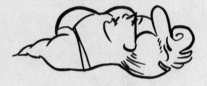

Rotate right

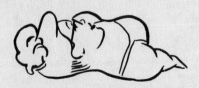

Rotate left

B-43

TO REDUCE THE BUST

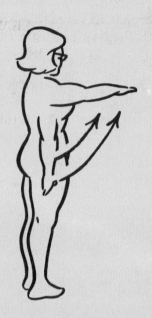

1. Toning up the muscles around the chest helps to eliminate fatty bust tissue and improve the bustline appearance. Stand erect and stretch your arms out at right angles to the body. Bring your arms forward level with your shoulders. Stretch your body upward as you breathe in. Relax and repeat ten to fifteen times.

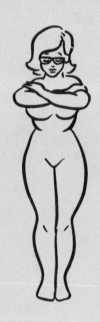

2. Fold your arms, clasping the biceps. As you raise your chest, raise your folded arms in an exaggerated manner and push against the clasped muscles of each arm.

TO REDUCE THE ARMS

1. Raise the shoulders in an exaggerated manner. Rotate each arm from the shoulders in a wide circular motion.

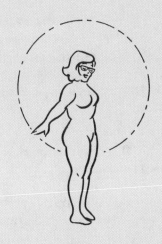

2. As you inhale, turn your hands backward and upward, bringing your fingers together. Exhale, relaxing hands and fingers. Repeat until tired.

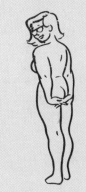

TO REDUCE THE WAIST

Waist exercises, and all twisting motions, are good to eliminate the fatty tissue which has accumulated around the waist and to strengthen the digestive organs as well.

1. Sit on the floor with the hands on the hips. Extend your legs far apart. Bend as far to the right as you can, over in front as far as you can, then bend to the left, and as far to

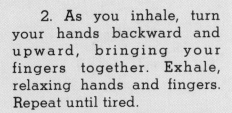

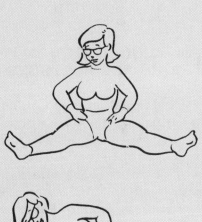

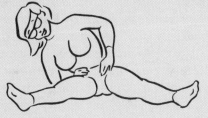

the back as you can. This movement is repeated in a rhythmic circular motion. Continue ten to twelve times. Relax completely before repeating.

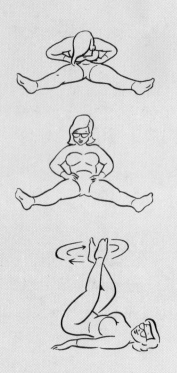

2. Lie flat on your back, on the floor or on your exercise board. Cross the ankles and pull the knees up over the abdomen. In this position, rotate the legs in a circular movement in as complete a circle as possible, bring the knees back to the original position each time. Repeat until fatigued. Relax completely before continuing in the opposite direction.

TO REDUCE THE HIPS, THIGHS AND BUTTOCKS

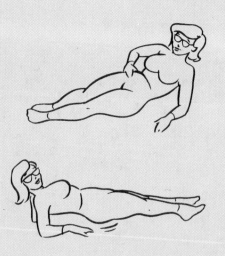

1. Lie flat on the floor, left or right side. Raise your body, resting on your elbow and hand. Bounce on the fleshy part of your thigh. Alternate your position to the other side and bounce. Then roll over on your back, resting on your elbows, and bounce on the fleshy part of your buttocks. Repeat a dozen times, each position. Relax completely and repeat.

2. Lie on a soft rug or blanket on the floor and lean on one elbow. Rub back and forth on the spot to be reduced about 20-30 times. Relax and continue procedure over a period of half an hour for the best results. Alternate this exercise by rolling the body on the floor as a barrel is rolled or clasp the knees and roll backward on the spine and forward on the hips.

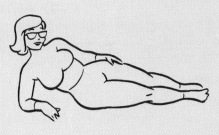

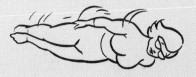

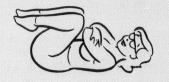

3. Lie flat on the floor. Bring the knees up to the abdomen. With the shoulders to the floor, and keeping the knees bent, roll to the right, slapping the right leg against the floor, the left leg slapping against the right leg. Repeat on the opposite side. Do this exercise about 50 times, then relax before repeating.

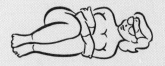

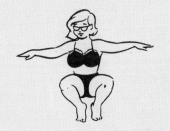

TO REDUCE THE LEGS AND ANKLES

1. For shapely legs and ankles, knee-bending combined with raising the body up on the toes, walking, running in place in your

room, slapping and brisk massage, and rotating the toes in a circular motion are all excellent.

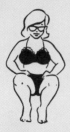

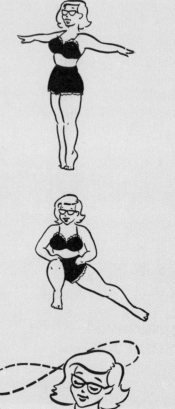

2. Assume a squatting position, keeping the back erect. Extend the right leg straight out to the side. Alternate position with the left leg. Increase the tempo as you grow more accustomed to this exercise.

Perhaps a note of caution should be mentioned here. You can get too much exercise, which is bad for the heart. All body movements should be in moderation, with plenty of relaxation. *Too much* exercise builds bulky muscles and an *APPETITE*.

For a lovely neck do figure eights

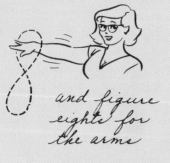

and figure eights for the arms

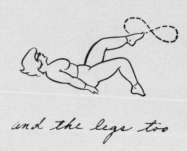

and the legs too

The best exercise for losing weight: Place both hands on the edge of the table and push away. Shaking the head "no" to offers of a second helping of food, and to too many starches and sweets, is another excellent reducing exercise that should be included on your **permanent** list of things to do to keep the body beautiful.

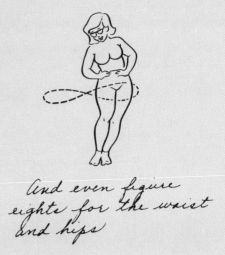

And even figure eights for the waist and hips

KEEPING THE POUNDS OFF IS AS IMPORTANT AS REDUCING THE POUNDS.

HOW TO MEASURE YOUR INCHES

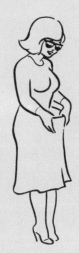

Keep up your "reducing morale" by measuring those vanishing pounds. But be fair, and measure your changes as they really are, just as a professional would. Hold the tape measure lightly around your bare body, stand easily, breathe naturally. Now you are ready to measure.

Neck. Measure the neck at the smallest portion.

Chin. Hold the tape measure under your chin and run the tape across the greatest protrusion, from ear to ear.

Upper Arm. Measure well up under the armpits and around the arms.

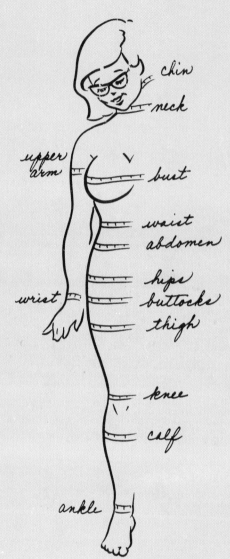

Wrist. Just below the wrist bone.

Bust. Run the tape across the point of your bust and around your back.

Waist. The smallest measurement around the middle of your body is your waist measurement. The waist should measure about ten inches less than your bust and hips.

Hips. Seven inches below your waist is where the hip measurement begins. The hips measure the same as your bust for a perfect figure measurement.

Buttocks. The largest masurement below the waist.

Abdomen. Run the tape around the hip bones, about an inch below the navel.

Thigh. Measure around the top of your leg or the "hump," which is both inside and outside of the leg.

Knees. Just above the knee joint.

Calf. The largest part of the lower leg.

Ankle. Just above the ankle bone.

Chapter 7

Your Bath

Cleanliness is indeed next to godliness and starts from within. Unless you have a clean skin with good tone, you cannot have the right eliminative activity, and without proper elimination, you cannot have "inner cleanliness" or the right mental attitude twoard yourself. Think of your bath as an aid to cleanliness and as an aid to good health as well

First, a warm, then a cool shower, is an invigorating start for the day. The full force of the spray is like the gentle prick of needles on the skin stimulating the body until it fairly glows with health. After you have turned down the warm water and the cooler water hits you, there is a moment when your breath will quicken. When you first begin to take the breath in sharply, that is the moment to complete your shower. Your reaction is good then. If you remain longer, the prolonged cold may be detrimental to your health. Avoid a cool or cold bath entirely if your vitality is low.

Warm baths relax aching muscles and tensed nerves, and have a soothing effect on the body, inducing sleep. Take your warm bath before retiring, both as an aid to relaxing sleep and to avoid body chills. Follow all intensive exercises with a warm water bath to relax the overworked muscles; then use a few, quick dashes of cold water to close the pores.

Too frequent tub baths and soaking in soapy water are poor ways to cleanse the body. When the pores are open, the skin may absorb the toxic wastes eliminating through the skin back into the pores again, as well as absorbing the soap in the water. Use less soap for body cleansing, and care should be taken to rinse all soap from the body to avoid clogging the pores. The best soaps are those made of natural ingredients, and your local health food store will most likely have a good selection. If you have skin problems, ask for a non-allergenic soap.

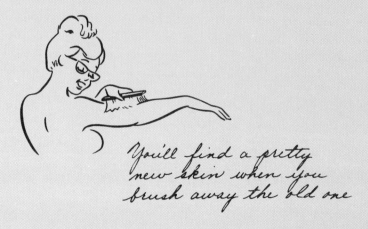

You'll find a pretty new skin when you brush away the old one

Daily dry friction brushing—or skin brushing—creates greater activity for the pores of the skin; is far more cleansing; elilminates more waste material than any soap and water bath, and the skin is not robbed of the natural oils needed to keep it from becoming too dry. Use a long-handled natural bristle brush as found in most health food stores. Use a dry Turkish towel if you prefer, but results are much more gratifying when a skin brush is used. You may dip the Turkish towel in cold water, wring out, and rub over the body vigorously. The friction rub, or the skin brush **BATH**, tones the skin, develops good circulation and aids in correcting mild skin conditions. The whole body is both stimulated and invigorated.

Sandow, the "Saxon Giant," who performed almost incredible feats of strength, had a skin of velvety softness that any women might envy. Part of his training to keep fit was the regular use of a hard, coarse vegetable bristle brush for dry skin bathing.

To become accustomed to the dry rub, brush softly at first. Avoid the more sensitive parts of the anatomy, and do not brush the face. Gradually increase the force of the brushing until your skin is comfortable at the amount of brushing it takes to create a soft pink blush effect. Avoid scrubbing too harshly, especially if your skin is delicate. You may use a soft brush on the face.

Use both face and body brushes without water. With the face brush, start at the forehead and work down over the eyes, along the nose, cheeks, chin, ears and finally, the neck, using a firm, brisk, rotary movement. With the body brush, brush the limbs with an upward movement or towards the heart, brushing the whole body gently at first until the skin becomes conditioned. Avoid brushing the breasts entirely. Devote at least three to five minutes, morning and night, to this type of bathing, and your skin—thus stimulated to better function—will actually become softer, your health will improve without question, and you will have lasting returns in both health and charm.

The daily air bath is a definite aid to good health, toning the skin and improving its texture. Body air baths, in the privacy of your own room, gradually build up your resistance to a cooler temperature and they may then be taken throughout the year.

Sunbathing is necessary to keep up the vitamins A and D content of the body. Vitamin D is necessary to control body calcium. For the average person, ten minutes a day is all that is needed. When more sun is taken, the body develops a suntan, a defense pigment that filters out the harmful rays of the sun. The body can absorb only so much vitamin D daily. Too much sun seriously affects the nervous system and lymph system, but a moderate amount of sun improves poor skin conditions and helps to eliminate skin blemishes.

Salt friction baths and Turkish towel baths, are both excellent for "toning" and are very exhilarating. But to overcome stagnant circulation, use the hot and cold foot baths. The alternating effect of hot and cold foot soaks, the temperature of the water not too extreme, wakes up a lagging bloodstream.

To help reduce your pounds, epsom salt baths may be taken once or twice a week, unless weakening. Use about 3 cups epsom salts to the average bath. Five to seven minutes is long enough or until the body has begun to perspire. Always follow these baths with a cold towel treatment, then with a brisk rubdown. The epsom salts, plus the water, eliminates toxic wastes as well as weight.

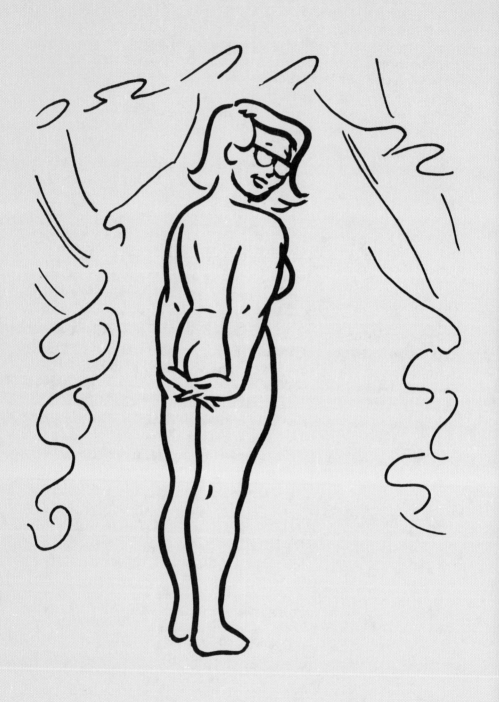

B-54

Steam baths or sauna baths are not harmful unless used immoderately and are a good means of eliminating toxic wastes from the system. As a means of reducing, they are only a partial measure. If you use these baths, use them along with an exercise and health diet routine for the best results. This type of bathing is best done under supervision.

Careful studies have shown us that water may be retained in the body to such an extent that the body weight will remain constant for some time, even when about half the daily food requirement has been taken. A daily weight score kept during this period may not show reduction in weight, but at the end of about 16 days, there may be a sudden loss of water from the tissues. Fatty tissue, as a rule, carries a high water content, and if the diet contains plenty of minerals and vitamins, some of this excess water and fat will be carried off by elimination. Drink vegetable broths instead of water for added minerals and vitamins during the reducing program.

Consider a bath as a worker of good health. The skin brush bath, the sunbath and the air bath are daily *MUSTS* in your health-building and weight-reducing program. All other baths you may choose are an added measure.

Chapter 8

Charm. . . The Natural Way

CHARM THE NATURAL WAY

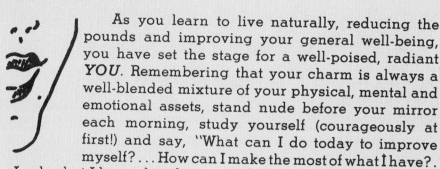 As you learn to live naturally, reducing the pounds and improving your general well-being, you have set the stage for a well-poised, radiant *YOU*. Remembering that your charm is always a well-blended mixture of your physical, mental and emotional assets, stand nude before your mirror each morning, study yourself (courageously at first!) and say, "What can I do today to improve myself?... How can I make the most of what I have?...Look what I have already accomplished!" Each day your self-esteem will grow a little stronger, for you are learning to play down your figure faults and to emphasize your strong points, and you have come a little closer to the sparkling, perfectly-poised person you want to be.

To help make a complete picture of glamour nature's way, the eyes must be sparkling, the hair lustrous, the smile attractive with whiter teeth, and the skin a skin you *really* love to touch. This chapter is devoted to many suggestions that will help you toward the attainment of these qualities.

THE EYES

The general health of the whole body must first be improved before you can improve on your eyes. A vitally alive bloodstream is necessary to keep the eye tissue in good order.

Along with correct foods, plenty of sleep is necessary to revitalize the eye muscles. Upon arising, spend a few moments bathing your eyes in cool water. Open them wide and close them tightly, holding them shut for a few moments, then open

and close them again. Repeat this exercise often throughout the day. Blinking the eyes is nature's way to relax tired and aching eye muscles when the eyes have not completely rested in sleep. Blink often to wake up sagging muscles and prevent bagginess. If you have been using your eye muscles but little in recent years, blink new warmth and lustre back into your eyes again. The wide-awake, animated eyes are young eyes.

To stimulate the internal flow of blood in and around the eyes, follow the fingers of one hand with both eyes while describing a large circle in front of the body. Allow the eyes to travel up and down and from side to side, as far as possible.

Lie down with the head lower than the feet, and follow an imaginary half circle with the eyes, without moving the head. Trace this imaginary half circle by allowing the eyes to travel to each side of the head, as far as possible. After tracing the upper half of the circle, trace the lower half. Repeat each exercise no more than a dozen times and rest the eyes by blinking them often.

Another exercise to assist in internal eye circulation is to hold a card with small lettering five inches away from the eyes, on a level with lettering on the wall which is large enough to read at a distance of twenty feet. Read the lettering five inches away, then lift the eyes and read the lettering twenty feet distant. By changing the focus of the lens of the eyes in this way, the lens is alternately made longer and shorter inducing a stepped-up, internal circulation.

Cover your right eye with your right hand, to close out all light. Look at a fairly bright light for a count of five with your left eye. Cover the eye for five counts, then uncover the eye to look at the light again for five counts. Repeat ten to a dozen times, and follow the same procedure with the right eye.

Train your eyes to read large and small print at a distance. Gradually reduce the size of print and each day lengthen the distance of vision.

Regular exercises are necessary to allow perfect circulation of blood to the eyes and the brain. Consistent practice of eye exercises may result in a change of glasses, if you wear them or in discarding them altogether.

  When the eyes have dust in them, use a pack of warm milk with a saturated watery solution of boric acid.

A drop of white sage honey diluted half-and-half with water and put into the eyes at night when retiring is both soothing and beneficial. Swimming, in clear water whenever possible, and horseback riding in nature's restful green playground are excellent cures for tired eyes. Nature knows that green has a soothing, restful effect on the eyes.

EXERCISE CHART FOR THE EYES

The eyes are important organs of the body and are fed by the bloodstream. A circulating and vitally alive bloodstream is necessary to keep the eye tissue in good working order. The toxicity of the intestinal tract affects the eyes and must therefore be attended to in all eye troubles.

Most people abuse their eyes too many hours a day. They rarely relax them. The average person uses his eyes twelve to sixteen hours a day constantly moving and focusing them on different objects.

WHEN THE EYES ARE TIRED, IT IS A GOOD SIGN THAT THE BRAIN AND NERVE SYSTEM IS TIRED ALSO, AND YOUR WHOLE BODY NEEDS A REST. THE EAGERNESS AND CONCENTRATED EFFORT THAT THE AVERAGE JOB DEMANDS OF THE EYES, KEEPING THE EYES ON ONE THING AT A SET DISTANCE FOR TOO

LONG DEMANDS THAT DURING SPARE HOURS WE USE OUR EYES DIFFERENTLY FROM THAT WHICH WE ARE ACCUSTOMED TO DOING DURING WORKING HOURS. TAKE CARE OF YOUR EYES BY HIKING AND LOOKING AT GREEN FIELDS. NATURE IS ALWAYS SOOTHING TO THE EYES. SWIMMING IN CLEAR COOL WATER AND HORSEBACK RIDING THROUGH PASTURES IS VERY SOOTHING TO THE EYES.

It has been said that we use eight times as much nervous energy through our eyes as any other organ in our body. The bright lights of the city; continual flicker of signs; reflections against our unnaturally colored buildings, walls, pavements, sidewalks, etc.; and automobile driving all focus our eyes in a strained position.

GENERAL HEALTH MUST BE IMPROVED TO IMPROVE THE EYES. AVOID OVERSTRAIN BY NOT USING THE EYES WHEN YOU ARE TIRED OR MENTALLY OVERWORKED. OUR DAY HAS BEEN INCREASED IN THE LAST DECADE BY THE ADVENT OF THE ELECTRIC LIGHT. BEFORE THIS WE WENT TO BED AT SUNDOWN.

THE BEST FOODS FOR THE EYES ARE: BARLEY WATER, OAT STRAW TEA, WHOLE RAW GOAT MILK, UNCOOKED GOAT MILK CHEESE (COW'S MILK FORBIDDEN), ROQUEFORT CHEESE, BLACKBERRY JUICE, VEAL JOINT BROTH, WHITE FISH THAT HAVE FINS AND SCALES, LEAFY TOPS OF VEGETABLES AND GRAPEFRUIT JUICE.

Plenty of sleep before twelve o'clock at night is good for the eyes as in most cases the cerebellum needs revitalizing.

A drop of white sage honey diluted with water put into the eyes at night when going to bed is helpful. When eyes have dust in them, use a pack of warm milk left on the eye with a saturated watery solution of boric acid.

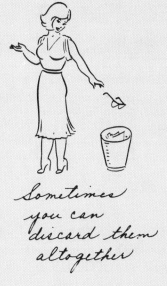

Sometimes you can discard them altogether

THE HAIR

The crowning glory of womanhood today is still the glory of beautiful hair. Lustrous, healthful hair is within the reach of everyone and is the key to the type of personality you wish to be.

The brightness and charm of your hair lies not only in grooming but in your general well-being. Nervous tension and emotional strain affect the condition of the hair just as seriously as will lack of certain foods in the daily diet.

Dry, brittle hair, very oily or greasy hair, is usually the result of diet deficiencies—lack of vitamins D and E, or a lack of iodine and silicon in the body. If your hair shows a tendency to be dull, dry or brittle, supplement the diet with foods high in silicon and iodine.

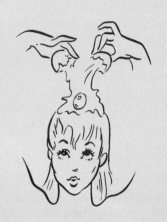

A few of the high iodine foods are: all seafoods, onions, garlic and pineapple.

High silicon foods are: oatstraw tea, barley, spinach, asparagus, lettuce, tomatoes, sprouts, figs, strawberries and watermelon.

Vitamin C may be found in the following: citrus fruits, melons, berries, apples, pineapple, tomatoes, cabbage, spinach, peas, broccoli, rutabaga, turnips and turnip greens, Brussels sprouts, celery, parsley, endive, watercress, cucumbers, cauliflower, radishes.

Some of the vitamin D foods are: fish oils and fish liver oils, egg yolk, butter and milk and green leafy vegetables.

Hair brushing is your insurance of healthy hair. Lie on a slanting exercise board or across the bed with the head hanging over the edge as you brush. Lie in this position daily for added stimulation to the scalp.

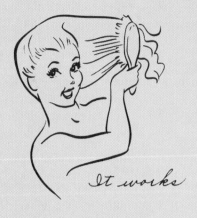

It works

Avoid the use of too stiff a brush on your sensitive scalp. Roll the hairbrush through the hair to give the hair shoots the right amount of exercise. Brush in the opposite direction from the way the hair grows, and in the way you part your hair, to increase the skin tone of the scalp. Massage the scalp for increased circulation and growth of hair.

Before shampooing, massage the scalp with the fingertips and brush the hair thoroughly. Make sure there is plenty of the natural oils in the shampoos you use. If you use a soap shampoo, a tincture of green soap, the castile soaps, apple pectin shampoo, coconut oil, jojoba or aloe vera shampoos are all good and less drying. Obtain a good lather by rubbing with a firm, even stroke and rinse. Add more soap for a second and even a third shampoo. Rinse the hair thoroughly, with a spray if possible, and add a lemon juice rinse to remove all traces of soap and to give a sheen to the hair. Dry in the air and sun, if possible. Air baths to the hair are just as important as air baths to the body. They give new life, stimulate new growth and promote beauty, but use discretion when exposing the hair to the intense rays of the sun. Over-exposure promotes dryness and fading of the hair coloring.

The egg shampoo does wonders in improving problem hair. After a brisk massage and head brushing, wrap hot towels, turban-wise, about your head, and leave on for about fifteen minutes. Remove the towels and massage the scalp. Repeat this process once again. To a diluted solution of liquid soap shampoo, add one whole egg. Wet the hair with lukewarm water and use half of the shampoo solution. Work well into the scalp. Rinse, avoiding too warm water, or the egg might curdle in the hair. After rinsing, repeat the entire process, using the other half of the egg shampoo solution. Finish with a lukewarm rinse and lemon juice. Thorough rinsing is absolutely necessary so that none of the egg is left on the hair or the hair will be sticky instead of fluffy. Dry with lintless towels and brush while drying. Rub a small amount of hair ointment into the scalp and brush in well.

If you are considering dyeing the hair, remember that this procedure may be harmful to your body. Many of the dyes are absorbed through the skin and sometimes cause kidney ailments or dermatitis. If the body is not healthy, if worried or angry or if menstruating, dyeing the hair during this time is especially dangerous. If you have a sensitivity to the particular kind of drug contained in the dye, the health of the entire body may be involved. In some cases, there has been a complete loss of hair.

Your personality is not vibrant or inviting if the harmony of tint in hair, skin and eyes does not have the appearance of naturalness. Govern the kind and frequency of shampoo and length of exposure to the sun, by the effect of each upon your own hair. Your diet, the amount of liquids consumed daily, and your general good health, all contribute greatly to the wide-awake appearance of your hair.

THE TEETH

You need good teeth to chew foods carefully and to prepare these foods for digestion and assimilation. Chewing the food well helps in the daily massage of the gums. Without healthy gums you cannot have healthy teeth. The fibrous foods, foods that are firm and resistant to chewing, are the best foods in the exercise of mastication. Chewing your food thoroughly helps you to build and retain strong, healthy teeth.

Though the teeth are white and harder than glass, they are still repaired and maintained by the bloodstream. Without the proper minerals in the blood to feed the teeth, decay is the

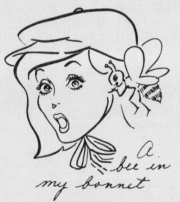

a bee in my bonnet

result. The greatest enemy of your teeth is white sugar and demineralized starches. These foods cause more tooth decay and infection than anything else. Pyorrhea, soft and bleeding gums, and all other oral troubles, are conditions you can help to eliminate by eating unrefined and vital foods. Fast living, little sleep, nerve strain, all deplete your alkaline reserve and produce an acid body caused by the breaking down of the chemical balance. An alkaline body is necessary to form good teeth.

Improve your teeth through the food you eat. Include greens daily and two glasses of fruit juice. The average bloodstream is usually depleted in calcium. This mineral is one of the elements necessary for sound teeth.

Some of the calcium foods are: raw milk, cheese, egg yolk, apricots, figs, prunes, cabbage, spinach, parsnips and tops of all vegetables, especially kale and beet greens. Raw milk is especially high in calcium and phosphorus. Raw pumpkin seeds, sunflower seeds, sesame seeds and nuts such as almonds are high in calcium. Fruits and vegetables, especially vegetables grown in the sunshine above the ground, have an abundance of calcium and other minerals necessary to retain good health and sound teeth. *(Refer to Mineral Chart in Appendix.)*

A clean, sweet mouth is the direct result of the simple, natural foods. An acid mouth is the result of eating refined sugars and starches. Cleanse your teeth daily, see your dentist regularly, follow the simple rules of eating natural foods, if you wish an attractive smile with strong, healthy teeth.

CLEANSING THE SKIN

The skin may be cleansed by applying apricot kernel oil, leaving it for a few minutes, then removing it with a dry washcloth. Lastly, rinse with cold water.

Since the skin is of such vital importance in maintaining internal health, we cannot overstress the value of its daily care. A beautiful skin is an active skin. The underlying muscles must be firm—firm through exercise, and they must be fed the proper nutrients from the blood. As you already know, a clean bloodstream is the direct result of a natural simple diet and proper elimination.

New skin underneath the old is ready to take its place as soon as the old drops off; but the skin underneath can be no better than the blood from which it is made. Your skin is most important to body elimination, eliminating more waste than either the lungs or kidneys. Fatty layers beneath the skin hinder this elimination.

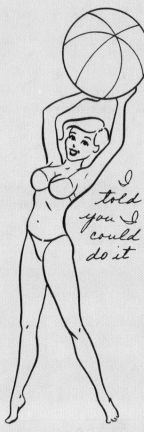

I told you I could do it

While reducing, remember it will take all of six months for the body muscle tone under the skin to fill in the wrinkles that may appear with the loss in weight. Diligent application of apricot oil will help prevent wrinkles from forming as you are taking off the pounds. Use no greasy chemicalized creams. Remember face creams do not *feed* the skin, but can harm it.

To tighten up the skin of the face and tone up the muscles, a local application of one teaspoon of epsom salts to one pint of water can be used once or twice a week. Apply hot wet towels that have been wrung from the epsom salts water. Leave the hot towels on the face until they begin to cool. Pinch the face slightly after these applications. Follow this procedure by applying an aloe vera lotion after the skin has cooled.

SAY!... LOOK AT OUR ANNIE NOW!

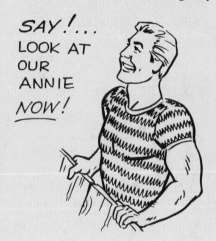

There are few skin conditions that cannot be improved if a natural living regimen is followed. Live the "health way" for a few months and note the difference in facial tone. Your natural coloring will return to your face and lips, and you will need to rely less and less on makeup to create the illusion of beauty. Natural living, including your daily skin brushing, will reduce the pores and the blackheads will disappear.

Some skin conditions are caused by nervous disorders, some by intestinal putrefaction and some by the daily physical and mental occupations. Go more than "skin deep" and take care of your internal organs first. Bring them to good health, and you will have both health and beauty from within. For a skin lotion, use aloe vera and apricot kernel oil. For a shampoo, you can use aloe vera and jojoba.

Sun and fresh air are important to good skin health, helping the pores to breathe more freely and increasing elimination. Intense rays of the sun are extremely injurious to the skin. The skin becomes dry and wrinkled, and serious skin troubles are often the result. The sun awakens the skin glands, as well as the internal glands, which release the pigment to tan, so avoid over exposure. Too much sun can be very injurious.

Clothing light in color is best for the skin, as dark clothing keeps out the beneficial rays of sun and light. Loose clothing and less of it allows the air to get to the skin.

Your looks are up to you. What you do about them is your business.

Chapter 9

Conclusion

The beauty we find *within* ourselves is the beauty everyone is seeking. You can attain this beauty and its outward expression through your own personal efforts.

Live in the joys you create. Make a friend of laughter and you will be loved, for to be loved and to be filled with love is the greatest thing in the world.

Be good to *YOU* and you will show a love for yourself, the most important person in the world.

Youth is joy. A joyous body is a young body. A good nature is a healthful nature for nature *IS* health. Let the glow of health come through and be "good natured" by filling yourself with the true joy of living. "Dis-harmony" and "dis-ease," including the acquired "dis-ease" of obesity, will fade away and the "new you" will begin in the mind and in the spirit.

You will find yourself. You can say, and say it with meaning, *"I feel wonderful!"* and know you have something to feel wonderful about, because you have the charm and the body to go with that feeling.

Be diligent and consistent in following the plan you have chosen as the plan best suited to your needs. Be patient and assured of its successful outcome, and soon your neighbors will stop you and say, "What have you done with yourself?"

Not only your friends, but your own mirror will tell you— *YOU WERE NEVER LOVELIER!*

Now I am
the person I always
wanted to be
and knew I
could be.

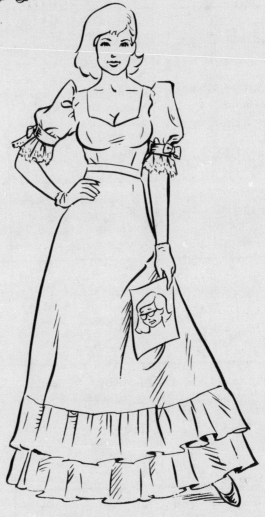

And what about you?

B-67

Appendix

MINERAL CHART
Chemical Element Analysis

Essential Mineral Salt	Mineral Salt Activity in the Body	Principle Sources
Calcium. Found and needed mostly in structural system. Tooth and bone mineral.	**Tone-Building in the Body.** Builds and maintains bone structure. Gives vitality, endurance. Heals wounds, counteracts acid.	Milk, cheese, raw egg yolk, apricots, figs, prunes, seeds, nuts, sprouts, cabbage, spinach, parsnips, lettuce, onions, dates, bran, tops of vegetables.
Chlorine. Found and needed mostly in the digestive system. Secretions.	**Cleanser in the Body.** Cleans. Expels waste. Freshens, Purifies. Disinfects.	Goat milk, cow milk, salt fish, cheese, cocoanut, beets, common salt, radishes.
Fluorine. Found and needed mostly in the structural system. Tooth enamel. Preserves bones.	**Disease Resister and Beautifier in Body.** Strengthens tendons. Knits bones.	Cauliflower, cabbage, cheese, raw goat milk, raw egg yolk, cod liver oil, Brussels sprouts, spinach, tomatoes, watercress.
Iodine. Found and needed mostly in nervous system. Gland and brain mineral.	**Metabolism Normalizer in Body.** Prevents goiter. Normalizes gland and cell action. Ejects and counteracts poisons.	Powdered Nova Scotia dulse and sea lettuce (very high), seafoods, carrots, pears, onions, tomatoes, pineapple, potato skin, cod liver oil, garlic, watercress.
Magnesium. Found and needed mostly in the digestive system. Nerve mineral. Nature's laxative.	**New Cell Promoter in the Body.** Relaxes nerves. Refreshes system. Prevents and relieves constipation and autointoxication.	Grapefruit, oranges, figs, whole barley, corn, wheat, cocoanut, goat's milk, raw egg yolk.

Essential Mineral Salt	Mineral Salt Activity in the Body	Principle Sources
Manganese. Found and needed mostly in nervous system. Tissue strengthener. Memory mineral.	**Controlling Nerves in the Body.** Increases resistance. Coordinates thought and action. Improves memory.	Nasturtium leaves, raw egg yolk, almonds, walnuts, watercress, mint, parsley, wintergreen, endive, pignolia nuts.
Phosphorus. Found and needed mostly in nervous system. Brain and bone mineral.	**Body and Nerve Builder in the Body.** Nourishes brain and nerves. Builds power of thought. Stimulates growth of hair and bone.	Seafoods, milk, raw egg yolk, parsnips, whole wheat, barley, yellow corn, nuts, peas, beans, lentils.
Potassium. Found and needed mostly in digestive system. Tissue and secretion mineral.	**Healer in the Body.** Liver activator. Strongly alkaline. Makes tissues elastic, muscles supple. Creates grace, beauty, good disposition.	Potato skin, dandelion, dill, sage, cress, dried olives, parsley, blueberries, peaches, prunes, cocoanut, gooseberries, cabbage, figs, almonds.
Silicon. Found and needed mostly in structural system. Nails, skin, teeth and hair.	**Surgeon in the Body.** Gives keen hearing, sparkling eyes, hard teeth, glossy hair. Tones system and gives resistance to the body.	Oats, barley, spinach, asparagus, lettuce, tomatoes, cabbage, figs, strawberries.
Sodium. Found and needed mostly in digestive system. Gland, ligament and blood builder.	**Youth Maintainer in Body.** Aids digestion. Counteracts acidosis. Halts fermentation. Purifies the blood.	Okra, celery, carrots, beets, cucumbers, string beans, asparagus, turnips, strawberries, oatmeal, cheese, raw egg yolk, cocoanut, black figs.

Essential Mineral Salt	Mineral Salt Activity in the Body	Principle Sources
Sulphur. Found and needed mostly in the nervous system. Brain and tissue mineral.	Purifies and Activates the Body. Purifies and tones the system. Intensifies feeling and emotion.	Cabbage, cauliflower, onions, asparagus, carrots, horseradish, shrimp, chestnuts, mustard greens.

Elimination & Slenderizing Regime

Take a hot bath every night during this diet regimen. Take an enema each day for the first four or five days, then discontinue and work for natural movements. Take nothing into the body for the first three days except water and fruit or vegetable juices, preferably grapefruit juice. Drink one glass of juice every four hours of each day. Eat ripe fruit and vegeteables only during the next two days, such as grapes, melons, tomatoes, pears, peaches, plums, baked apple. Dried fruits soaked overnight in boiling water, such as prunes, figs and peaches, are especially good.

During the following six days, the breakfasts consist of fresh fruit. Between breakfast and lunch any other kind of fruit may be eaten. For lunch, have a salad of three to six vegetables—some leafy—and two cups of potato peeling broth (directions follow). For dinner, eat two or three steamed vegetables and two cups of vital broth. Squash are the most filling low-calorie vegetables. If hungry between meals or before retiring, eat fruit or drink fruit juice.

Potato Peeling (or Potassium) Broth

2 C. celery tops
1/2 C. chopped parsley
3 C. celery stalks
1 carrot, diced
2 C. potato peelings (1/2" thick—
do not use the rest of the
potato)

1 onion, diced
1 tsp Savita or Vegex
seasoning
2-1/2 qt water (distilled)

Finely chop all vegetables. Bring slowly to a boil. Simmer approximately 20 minutes. Strain, using only the liquid.

This elimination regimen may be followed whenever a general weight reduction is desired, or if your skin breaks out, whenever a cold appears or if constipation is present, and as a general body cleanser two or three times a year.

THE WEIGHT-WATCHER'S CHART

Month	1st Week	2nd Week	3rd Week	4th Week	Monthly Total
January					
February					
March					
April					
May					
June					
July					
August					
September					
October					
November					
December					

Total Number of Pounds Lost During Your Reducing Program:

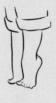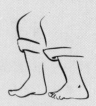

FOOT EXERCISES

These foot exercises will help callouses, fallen arches (both mertatarsal and longitudinal), cramps in toes and legs, weak ankles, flat feet, bunions, corns and other troubles.

1. Raise leg forward and up stretching the point of toe downward.

2. Spread toes apart as far as possible, and roll front arch on a golf ball.

3. Stand on a book or stairs and bend toes downward.

4. Raise up on toes while standing or walking.

5. Walk on outside edge of feet.

6. Grasp marbles under toes, pick up and drop marbles into a vessel.

7. For shapely ankles, put leg forward and move toes in a circular motion toward inside.

8. Put one foot in front of the other and bend straight down. Keep heel of back foot on floor.

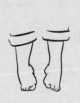

HOW TO MAKE A SLANTING BOARD

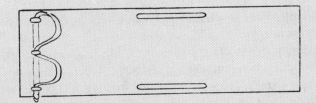

The board is 18 inches to 20 inches wide, 6 feet long, of 5-ply wood 3/4-inches thick. Side handles are made by cutting 3/4 of an inch in from edge, 24 inches from head end of board. The slot is 1-inch wide and 18-inches long. A strap fastened near the foot end holds ankles to keep the body from sliding and to bring the body to a sitting position when exercising. (See other section of this book for directions and pictures of slanting board exercises.)

A Note of Sincerity

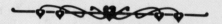

I feel there is one thing above all others that you wouldn't want me to do, and that is to fool you. I wouldn't want anyone to fool me either. That is why I have made this book as accurate and honest as I can.

This book presents a program which, if sincerely followed, will add to your health, vitality, beauty, work efficiency, mental attitude and positive feelings about yourself. This is what I can promise you from my end.

Will you meet me at my level of sincerity? Will you promise to give my program an honest try?

My obligation is to do the right thing for you. You also have an obligation to do right by me and my program. I feel an attitude of sincerity is one of the most important requirements for making this program work for you.

You must realize that 95% of our weight problems have come from diets—imbalanced eating. You need to get off diets once and for all, and that is my purpose in this program.

Here, I am showing you a healthy way to live. Once You are using foods properly and living right, you won't need diets. You'll look and feel wonderful without them.

—Bernard Jensen, Ph.D.

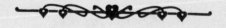

For Your Good Health—
The Writings of Dr. Jensen

Build a Library of Right Living—Look for Dr. Jensen's many books sharing the natural principles of happy, healthy living. If they are not available in your local bookstore or health food store, you may order direct from the address below.

Food Healing for Man—A wonderful primer of nutrition and food facts for everyone, especially for those starting out in the nutrition field, exploring the role of deficiencies in disease and the restorative power of a balanced food regimen.

The Healing Mind of Man—Wholistic healing principles for the body, mind and spirit, including the roles of inspiration, wisdom, peace and beauty in healing. The many stories here from Dr. Jensen's experience will not only uplift but delight readers.

World Keys to Health and Long Life—Secrets of health and longevity from around the world, collected in Dr. Jensen's journeys to over 55 countries of the world, visiting the oldest people on earth, including the Hunzas, the Caucasus mountain people of Russia, the strong old men of Turkey, the long-lived Rumanians and the Vilcabambains of Ecuador.

Creating A Magic Kitchen—How to turn your kitchen into a magic place where health and vitality flow into the entire family.

Vital Health from Your Kitchen—Many recipes and convenient menu plans to put you and your family on the path of healthful living.

A New Lifestyle for Health and Happiness—How to begin living a more natural lifestyle to prevent disease and enhance well-being in an age of fast living, stress and anxiety.

OTHER BOOKS BY DR. JENSEN: *Breathe Again Naturally, How to Deal with Catarrh, Bronchitis, Asthma; Survive This Day; Blending Magic; Doctor-Patient Handbook; Tissue Cleansing Through Bowel Management.* **WRITE FOR FULL LIST AND PRICES.**

THE SPOKEN WORD OF DR. JENSEN—His Best Lectures
(60-90 minute cassette tapes)

Dr. Jensen's entire Nutrition Course is available on tape: *Nutrition I, Nutrition II* and *Clinical Nutrition*, each set 10 hours.

The Chemical Story, Building a Better Way to Eat, Replacement Therapy, Regularity Management, Key to Inner Calm, Nature Has a Remedy, and many more. **Three Latest Tapes:** *Food Healing for Man, Nutrition for Longevity* and *Nutrition for Youth*. **WRITE FOR FULL LIST AND PRICES.**

VIDEO TAPES OF DR. JENSEN'S TALKS

At last, available in VHS and BETA. Dr. Jensen's greatest lectures before live audiences.

Rejuvenation Program: American Series: 5 tapes, including **The Healing Mind of Man, The Chemistry of Man** and **Nature Has a Remedy,** recorded "live" in California.

Joy of Living: Australian Series— 9 tapes, including **Nutrition for Youth, Vital Foods for Total Health** and **Food Healing for Man (I & II),** recorded "live" in Brisbane, Australia.

World Search for Health and Long Life— Dennis Weaver narrates this beautiful "around the world" health adventure with Dr. Jensen.

Tissue Cleansing—Three hours of Dr. Jensen's teachings on colon health, so important in today's world, including one tape on *Tissue Cleansing* and one tape on *Nutrition.*

For further information on books, cassette tapes, video tapes and prices, write to:

DR. BERNARD JENSEN
Route 1, Box 52
Escondido, CA 92025